WARM CLIMATES AND WESTERN MEDICINE: THE EMERGENCE OF TROPICAL MEDICINE, 1500–1900

THE WELLCOME INSTITUTE SERIES IN THE HISTORY OF MEDICINE

Forthcoming Titles

Marshall Hall: 1790–1857: Science and Medicine in Early Victorian Society
Diana Manuel

The Correspondence of James Jurin (1684–1750): Physician and Secretary of the Royal Society
Andrea Rusnock

History of Cardiology
P. Fleming

Fantasy Surgery
Ann Dally

Operative Chymist: A Biography of Thomas N. R. Morson
Anthony F. P. Morson

Academic inquiries regarding the series should be addressed to the editors W. F. Bynum and Roy Porter at the Wellcome Institute for the History of Medicine, 183 Euston Road, London NW1 2BE, UK

WARM CLIMATES AND WESTERN MEDICINE: THE EMERGENCE OF TROPICAL MEDICINE, 1500–1900

Edited by David Arnold

Amsterdam - Atlanta, GA 1996

First published in 1996
by Editions Rodopi B. V., Amsterdam – Atlanta, GA 1996.

Design and Typesetting by Christine Buckley, the Wellcome Trust.
Printed and bound in The Netherlands by Editions Rodopi B. V.,
Amsterdam – Atlanta, GA 1996.

British Library Cataloguing in Publication Data
A catalogue record for this book is available from the British Library
ISBN 90-5183-923-5 (Bound)

Warm
Warm Climates and Western Medicine: The Emergence of Tropical Medicine, 1500–1900 ed. by David Arnold – Amsterdam – Atlanta, GA: Rodopi. – ill.
(Clio Medica 35 The Wellcome Institute Series in the History of Medicine)

CIP-GEGEVENS KONINKLIJKE BIBLIOTHEEK, DEN HAAG

Front cover: Sassoon General Hospital, Poona, India: a queue of patients awaiting treatment. Wood engraving by CR,
By kind permission of the Wellcome Institute Library, London

Met index, lit. opg.
ISBN 90-5183-923-5 (Bound)
Trefw.: geneeskunde; tropen; geschiedenis.

Printed in The Netherlands

Contents

Acknowledgements

With the exception of the essay by Julyan Peard, earlier versions of the essays in this volume were presented at a Wellcome Symposium on 'Tropical Medicine Before Manson: Warm Climates and Western Medicine, *c.*1500–1900', held in London on 25–26 March 1993. The Editor wishes to thank the Wellcome Trust for its financial and organizational support for this meeting, and Frieda Houser and Sally Bragg of the Wellcome Institute for their administrative assistance. Particular thanks are due to Bill Bynum at the Wellcome Institute for his enthusiastic support, his very considerable help in planning and running the symposium and his help in preparing this volume for the press. A word of thanks, too, to the other participants in the symposium, especially to Guenter Risse, for his paper on hospitals in sixteenth-century Mexico.

Notes on Contributors

David Arnold is Professor of South Asian History at the School of Oriental and African Studies, London. He edited *Imperial Medicine and Indigenous Societies* (1988), and is the author of *Colonizing the Body: State Medicine and Epidemic Disease in Nineteenth-Century India* (1993).

Peter Boomgaard is Director of the Royal Institute of Linguistics and Anthropology in Leiden. He has published a number of articles on the demographic, medical and environmental history of Indonesia from the late eighteenth century and a book entitled *Children of the Colonial State: Population Growth and Economic Development in Java, 1795–1880* (1989).

Philip D. Curtin is Herbert Baxter Adams Professor of History at Johns Hopkins University and has written extensively on disease and medicine in the context of Europe overseas. Among his major works are *The Image of Africa: British Ideas and Action, 1780–1850* (1964), and *Death by Migration: Europe's Encounter with the Tropical World in the Nineteenth Century* (1989).

Mark Harrison is currently at the School of Cultural Studies, Sheffield Hallam University and is working on a history of the Army Medical Corps. His published work includes *Public Health in British India: Anglo-Indian Preventive Medicine, 1859–1914* (1994) and several articles on public health in nineteenth-century India.

Douglas M. Haynes is an Assistant Professor in the Department of History, Unversity of California, Irvine. He was awarded his Ph.D. from the University of California, Berkeley, in 1992, for a dissertation entitled, 'From the Periphery to the Center: Patrick Manson and the Development of Tropical Medicine as a Medical Specialty in Britain, 1870–1900'.

Kenneth F. Kiple teaches in the Department of History, Bowling Green State University, Ohio, and has written widely on the medical history of the West Indies, including *The Caribbean Slave: A Biological History* (1984). He has also edited *The African Exchange: Towards a Biological History of Black People* (1987) and *The Cambridge World History of Human Disease* (1993).

Anne Marie Moulin is Director of Research at CNRS, INSERM, Paris. She has worked on the history of the Pasteur Institutes and Pastorian medicine in Africa and the Middle East.

Kriemhild Coneè Ornelas teaches sociology and anthropology at Bowling Green State University, Ohio. She has published essays on the 'Columbian Exchange' and the 'African Exchange' and is co-editor of the Cambridge History and Culture of Human Nutrition Project.

Michael A. Osborne teaches history of science and environmental studies at the University of California, Santa Barbara. He is currently at work on a history of French tropical medicine. His most recent book is *Nature, the Exotic and the Science of French Colonialism* (1994).

Julyan G. Peard teaches in the Department of History, San Francisco State University. Her Ph.D. thesis on 'The Tropicalista School of Medicine of Bahia, Brazil, 1860–89', for Columbia University, was completed in 1990.

M. N. Pearson is Professor of History, University of New South Wales. Among his books are *Merchants and Rulers in Gujarat* (1976); *The Portuguese in India* (1987), and *Pious Passengers: The Hajj in Earlier Times* (1987). He is currently working on various aspects of the medical interaction between India and Europe in the early modern period.

Michael Worboys is Wellcome Reader in the History of Medicine at Sheffield Hallam University. His main research interest is in the history of science and British imperialism, on which he has published several articles. He is currently completing a study of germ theories and bacteriology in the period 1870–1940.

Introduction: Tropical Medicine before Manson

David Arnold

Manson and the Making of Tropical Medicine

It is always historically suspect to define a period of history in terms of what followed after it – pre-Columbian, pre-industrial, pre-Mansonian – as if the generations who happened to be born before Columbus, the Industrial Revolution or Patrick Manson lived in impenetrable darkness or wasted their lives in messianic expectation. And yet, with respect to the history of tropical medicine, such is the picture commonly presented to us. It was, and perhaps largely remains, the conventional wisdom that tropical medicine only emerged as a medical specialty in the final decade or so of the nineteenth century and that before that time Western medical practice in the tropics constituted little more than a 'rudimentary field of medicine'.[1]

H. H. Scott, in his *History of Tropical Medicine,* first published in 1939 but still widely cited, referred somewhat condescendingly to the 'vague, empirical ideas' and to the 'curious mingling of acute observation and vague surmise' that characterized the understanding of disease causation in the tropics before the end of the eighteenth century. Only after that time did he detect 'the beginnings of rational thought' and an attempt to 'consider the problems scientifically'. This movement eventually, in Scott's view, found its fullest expression in the work of Patrick Manson and his great achievement, the founding of the London School of Tropical Medicine in 1899.[2] While more sceptical than Scott about the validity of tropical medicine as a discrete field of scientific enquiry and medical practice, many modern scholars have nonetheless adopted a chronology that similarly emphasizes Manson and the 1890s in the emergence of tropical medicine. In his recently published study of bilharzia, John Farley has gone so far as to argue that it was only in 1898, after 300 years of activity overseas, that the British finally 'declared war on tropical diseases'. They did so, he suggests, as a result of two compelling causes – firstly, the germ theory of disease, which suggested that disease in tropical regions was not specifically linked to climate and could, therefore, be overcome by medical science, and, secondly, the concurrent expansion of the British Empire into new tropical territories, especially in Africa. Manson's timely appeal for support for tropical medicine attracted the politically powerful backing of Joseph Chamberlain, the Secretary of State for the Colonies, and barely a year later the London School of Tropical medicine came into being. This helped to establish the scientific respectability of tropical medicine and provided both model and stimulus for similar schools, institutes and associations around the world.[3] Manson, almost single-handedly, it would seem, had 'invented the idea of tropical diseases as a distinct group of afflictions' and transformed a 'rudimentary field of medicine' into a highly prestigious and politically influential 'scientific specialty'.[4]

There have, of course, been those who have questioned Manson's exclusive right to be honoured as the founder of tropical medicine. Pasteur, Laveran and Koch might reasonably claim a share of the credit, and the list of luminaries has at one time or another been extended to include such pioneers as Grassi, Ross, Finlay and Reed, depending in part upon the nationality of the author.[5] There were also those among Manson's contemporaries who wondered what was new about his tropical medicine that had not been taught at the Army Medical School at Netley since the 1860s, or particularly desirable about locating a School of Tropical Medicine in London rather than in the tropics themselves.[6]

There have been other dissenters, too, writers whose aim was less to belittle Manson and his achievements than to acknowledge the contributions made by many other Western doctors to the study of tropical diseases from at least the early eighteenth century onwards. In his Presidential Address as Director of the London School of Hygiene and Tropical Medicine in 1925, Andrew Balfour stated that it was 'quite wrong to speak of Patrick Manson as the "Father of Tropical Medicine". He was the Father, most undoubtedly, of *modern* Tropical Medicine', but behind him stood a long line of British and American pioneers. Balfour's genealogy began with the eighteenth-century army physician Sir John Pringle and his naval counterpart James Lind, and continued with British medical writers like Hillary and Moseley in the West Indies and the American Benjamin Rush in Philadelphia, and East India 'surgeons' of the early nineteenth century, such as Annesley, Ballingall and Twining.[7] But typically accounts such as this do not seek to place eighteenth- or nineteenth-century physicians in the intellectual, social and political context of their own times, as today's historian of medicine might do. Rather they cast a retrospective glance from the high ground of the twentieth century over the earlier travails of medicine in the tropics, commending some individuals for their scientific prescience, reproving others for their shameful ignorance and simple-minded pursuit of false trails. As H. W. Mulligan remarked specifically of British medical writers in India: 'The published works of these and other pioneer investigators of tropical diseases did much to define the problems and, in some cases, to highlight the astute observations that, many years later, were proved to be well founded.'[8]

But, the palm of honour for being 'the father of tropical medicine' has nonetheless usually gone to Patrick Manson – more for his role in establishing the London School than for his filariasis research in China 20 years earlier – and that title was bestowed on him even in his own lifetime.[9] Manson himself laid out the rationale for tropical medicine as he understood it in an address given to students at St George's Hospital in London in October 1897. He advanced two main claims for 'special education in tropical medicine' in Britain. One was that the country had become the centre of 'a great and growing tropical empire'. The other was that because tropical disease was 'in many respects ... widely different from the diseases of temperate climates', 'special knowledge' was needed for their diagnosis and successful treatment. Of the 'dozens of diseases more or less special to the tropics', Manson cited malaria ('eminently a tropical disease'), beriberi, filariasis and ankylostomiasis. Although, he said, more than a fifth of British and Irish medical graduates practised in 'warm climates' (or, as members of the armed forces, were liable to do so), tropical medicine was virtually ignored in British medical education. It was, therefore, in his view, imperative, especially in view of the expansion of the empire and the recent advances in 'tropical pathology' that 'this vast army of medical men should be properly equipped for their special work'.[10]

Having thus defined the subject and its importance, Manson then went on to consolidate his leadership in the field by establishing the London School of Tropical Medicine and by publishing in 1898 his *Tropical Diseases: A Manual of the Diseases of Warm Climates.* This, it has been said, 'set out the rubrics of the new discipline of tropical medicine',[11] but it might also be noted that, despite Manson's bold claims for his subject, the second half of the book's title in effect invoked the medicine of an earlier age. It is this pre-Mansonian age of 'warm climates' and Western medicine that this volume of essays seeks to investigate, both in its own right and in order to establish its connections with the newer tropical medicine that was emerging by the 1880s and 1890s.

It has increasingly been argued that the idea of tropical medicine is in many respects anomalous, if not erroneous. It is the only medical specialty defined by relation to a specific geographical area, and is founded on a dubious distinction (as even a cursory review of the history of Manson's 'eminently' tropical disease, malaria, would suggest) between the diseases of tropical and temperate areas. Many so-called tropical diseases are not inherently confined to the tropics, though they may now have been banished from more temperate lands. They are, in practice, diseases of poverty, social deprivation, malnutrition and insanitary conditions.[12] It is nonetheless possible to argue that a cluster of closely related developments marked out the last decade or two of the nineteenth century as being of revolutionary significance in relation to medicine in the tropics. There were major advances in the emerging scientific disciplines of bacteriology and parasitology (including helminthology, protozoology and medical entomology), as well as in the allied fields of microscopy and immunology. Alongside this was the innovative combination of laboratory research and experimentation (often conducted in metropolitan institutes) with field observations in tropical countries, and the targeting of specific diseases (notably malaria, but also sleeping sickness and yellow fever) for both laboratory research and public health campaigns. Driven by the political and economic imperatives of the 'new imperialism', there was also rapidly growing interest in diseases affecting indigenous peoples – as a factor both in furthering European health and in the profitable exploitation of labour.[13]

Establishing the antecedents of Mansonian tropical medicine in the ideas and practices of the earlier part of the nineteenth century, or, alternatively, demonstrating the nature and causes of the change that occurred in the creation of the new tropical medicine of the 1890s, are tasks on which historians are already embarked, and some of those questions are pursued further in several essays here. What was different about the tropical medicine of the late nineteenth century? What was carried over from the old medicine of 'warm climates' into the new tropical medicine? What attempts were made outside Europe (in India, Algeria or Brazil) to reconcile the older discourses of body humours and environmental miasmas with the new language of microbes and germs? When were Hippocrates and Galen finally laid to rest? When were Pasteur and Manson installed as the new orthodoxy?

But there are a number of other reasons to reopen the file on pre-Mansonian tropical medicine. One is that it is timely. It is now almost 100 years since the founding of the London and Liverpool schools of tropical medicine in 1899, and if it is just over 500 years since Columbus blundered into the Americas, it is also close to a half-millennium since Vasco da Gama breezed into the Indian Ocean. Anniversaries pall, but these dates do at least remind us of the four centuries of Europe's medical involvement with Africa, Asia and the Americas before Manson and of the ways in which historians working in other parts of the discipline are beginning to rethink the nature of that complex and multi-faceted encounter. Those 400 years represent a vast expanse of time and a huge geographical area for which – with a few notable exceptions, particularly in the pioneering work of Philip Curtin[14] – we have remarkably little informed and critical scholarship. Now that we know much more about the earlier history of medicine in Europe itself, now that we are no longer governed by the kinds of teleological assumptions and narrowly 'scientific' criteria of previous generations of medical historians, it is possible to approach the pre-Mansonian history of Europe's medicine overseas from a number of fresh perspectives. Moreover, now that we have several studies which have re-examined European medicine overseas during the high imperial period from the 1880s to the 1920s,[15] it is all the more imperative that we look back to an earlier age and reassess its place in medical history.

Inventing Tropicality

If we construe tropical medicine in terms of specific scientific developments, discoveries and personalities – the germ theory of disease, the new understanding of filariasis, malaria, kala-azar and yellow fever, the role of Patrick Manson in establishing tropical medicine as a metropolitan specialty – then there is an obvious sense in which this was the creation, even the invention, of the period 1890 to 1910. But if we understand tropical medicine in a wider sense, as the specialist medicine of 'warm climates' and 'torrid zones', equipped with its own literature and practitioners, and if we see it as an integral part of the way in which Europeans perceived and sought to gain control over a large part of the globe, then it has a much longer history, reaching back to the earliest years of European exploration and conquest. Indeed, medicine was a conspicuous element in the process of European exploration and colonization virtually from the outset – in the search for medicinal herbs and spices, in the struggle to stay alive in new lands, in the manner in which the newcomers exchanged or extracted knowledge, healing goods and therapeutic services in places as far apart as Mexico, India, Java and Japan.

In this longer-term perspective on tropical medicine the issues are not just about constructing a chronology of scientific discovery, or about faltering progress towards a twentieth-century (and Western) understanding of disease. Rather the questions relate to the place of Europe's medicine in the wider world and how that world came, over time, to be demarcated and defined. The issues relate to the nature and status of medical practitioners and their patients, to the role of physicians as colonial, rather than simply medical, experts and observers, to long-term attitudes to indigenous societies and cultures, and to environments geographically distant and culturally remote from those of Europe itself. Such a history is not only of value in locating medical ideas and practices in the texts and contexts of their own time rather than at the wrong end of teleology's telescope. It also helps to establish more clearly the nature of the interaction with other cultures and environments and the changing nature of medical responses to, and conceptualizations of, other lands.

Two characteristics of this early tropical medicine seem to stand out. The first was a sense of 'otherness' attached by Europeans to warm countries and tropical places. This sense of difference was reflected in accounts of plants, animals, climate and topography, and in descriptions of indigeneous societies and cultures, but (perhaps because physicians were significant and scientifically informed observers) it was particularized through the discussion of disease. The second characteristic was the power of localism, manifested through the particular medical needs and social composition of the local inhabitants, the impact of indigenous practitioners on Western traders and travellers, the use of local drugs and different topographies to counter disease, the growth of local medical services and even local schools of thought and practice. All of these remained closely tied to developments in medical ideas, training and professional status in Europe itself, but they also in various ways helped to define the medicine of 'warm climates' in contradistinction to the metropolis, with its ignorance of local conditions and lack of local expertise.

Let us begin with 'otherness'. To do this we need to understand the tropics as a conceptual, and not just physical, space.[16] What was it that justified the notion of 'the tropics'? I would argue that calling a part of the globe 'the tropics' (or by some equivalent term, such as the 'torrid zone') was a Western way of defining something culturally and politically alien, as well as environmentally distinctive, from Europe and other parts of the temperate zone.

It may well be that this sense of difference was not initially very prominent in the minds of European travellers. During the first voyage to the Caribbean, Columbus made repeated comparisons between the trees, birds and fish he saw there and those he knew in Spain – some seemed familiar, others utterly strange – and historians have commented on the way in which Europe only gradually came to recognize how different the New World was from the Old.[17] The first European impressions – or expectations – often inclined more to the paradisical than the pestilential, and only slowly did a more negative and alarming concept of the tropics emerge. Thus early in the seventeenth century Sir Walter Raleigh remarked in his *History of the World* that, whether or not Paradise and perpetual spring were located in 'the Tropicks' as many believed, they certainly held 'the fearfull and dangerous thunders and lightnings, the horrible and frequent earthquakes, the dangerous diseases, the multitude of venimous beasts and wormes'.[18]

A century or so after Raleigh, and particularly from the mid-eighteenth century onwards, this kind of negative, or at least exotic, representation of the tropics was becoming relatively common in medical literature, especially in relation to West Africa and the West Indies. Writers like the Dutchman Bosman on the Guinea Coast and the Englishmen Hunter and Moseley in the West Indies repeatedly stressed the fierce malevolence of the tropics – the sudden hurricanes and devastating storms, the tigers onshore matched by predatory sharks at sea, and, by extension or by analogy, the extreme violence of tropical diseases compared to those of Europe.[19] Although 'intemperance', 'venery', and imprudent dress, diet and demeanour among new arrivals might add to their vulnerability to disease, the tropical climate was almost universally considered to be the prime cause of European ill health and to distinguish the diseases of 'warm climates' from those of the temperate zone. The heat, humidity and rapid temperature changes of the tropics were thought to have a grievous effect on European constitutions, to predispose to disease, even where they did not actually cause it, just as the abundant and tiresome insects, the rapid processes of putrefaction and decay, and the offensive smells of swamps and rotting vegetation added to the acute, indeed palpable, sense of tropical danger. The hot, wet tropics produced deadly miasmas on a scale, and of an intensity, unmatched in Europe. In the 'torrid zone' disease 'put on a different aspect and character': it ran its course rapidly and violently, and so called for exceptionally drastic and speedy remedies.[20]

The great reverence paid by eighteenth- and early nineteenth-century writers to Hippocrates – 'that wise Father and Prince of Physicians'[21] – strengthened this belief in the singular dangers of tropical airs, waters and places compared to their temperate counterparts, especially in steamy jungles, swamps and deltas, though some writers significantly noted the absence of such diseases as yellow fever from the Hippocratic corpus and placed greater reliance on Arab and Persian authorities, like Rhazes, for their observations of diseases (like elephantiasis) more common to warmer climates.[22]

But it was not the Hippocratic revival and miasmatic theory alone that, from about the mid-eighteenth century onwards, sharpened the sense of there being something distinctive about tropical diseases and medicine in the tropics. Several practical considerations were also involved. The increased involvement of European traders, soldiers and sailors in West Africa, the West Indies, and latterly in India, gave added urgency to the investigation of diseases seen to be peculiar to the tropics or to exist there in more extreme forms than in Europe. The trans-Atlantic slave trade and the plantation economies of the Caribbean were a major stimulus; so, too, were heavy troop losses in the West Indies during the Seven Years War and the French Revolutionary and Napoleonic wars.[23] The arguments about the ability of Europeans to survive and settle in the tropics that were being so earnestly debated in Manson's day in the light of the germ theory of disease had been extensively discussed a century earlier on the islands of the West Indies and in the forts and 'factories' of maritime Asia. Scores of writers, whether local practitioners or mere sojourners in the service of their country's army or navy, capitalized on this new-found interest by publishing their own account of the diseases of 'hot climates', stressing their own expertise and chiding the ignorance of their fellow physicians.[24]

In many of these late eighteenth- and early nineteenth-century accounts can be found another distinguishing feature of this emerging literature – a discussion of the diseases and medical practices of indigenous, or (in the case of the West Indies) slave, populations. In some instances, the motive was little more than ethnographical curiosity. More often it was driven by concern for the health and hence the productive capacity of plantation workers, or the risks of 'native' diseases infiltrating white households. The vulnerability of Europeans as 'exotics', constitutionally and temperamentally ill-suited to the tropics, 'uprooted' from the environment that had (in the age of Montesquieu) supposedly shaped their frame and character, or, by contrast, the greater adaptability of indigenes, their physiologies and folkways, introduced an important geographical and cultural dynamic into the discussion of disease causation, transmission and susceptibility. Even when Western medicine did not address their needs directly, the non-whites continually informed the Western understanding of the tropics and of tropical diseases – as clinical objects, as sources of epidemic danger, as sick or 'shirking' workers. This combination of unfamiliar peoples and alien places helped define the identity and distinctive preoccupations of the medicine of 'hot countries'.[25]

Three other developments of the late eighteenth and early nineteenth centuries, though clearly attributable to Europe, further established the distinctiveness of tropical climates and diseases. One was the increasingly confident use of statistics to illustrate patterns of European mortality and the impact of specific diseases. Until the early 1800s medical writers tended to present their data in the form of narratives, describing the epidemics that had afflicted a territory over a period of years, especially in relation to climate and seasons, but with only an impressionistic notion of the number and type of fatalities that had occurred. By the 1820s, 1830s and 1840s, however, medical writers were making extensive use of data, sometimes giving figures for morbidity as well as mortality and often in tabular form, priding themselves on their new statistical sense.[26] This was, of course, a development shared with the medicine of temperate Europe and North America, but it had a particular significance for tropical medicine in isolating and providing 'scientific' evidence for the extraordinarily high levels of white mortality in the tropics compared to Europe, and the extreme vulnerability of certain groups like soldiers and sailors, especially when comparable statistics for indigenous groups were lacking. Of course, as Philip Curtin reminds us, medical statistics could be both grossly misleading and highly influential at the same time.[27] But the general effect as far as the early nineteenth century was concerned was to give a statistical and scientific specificity to the hitherto generalized dangers of tropical climates and to encourage measures to combat them.

A parallel development was the growth of medical geography and topographical surveys, again along lines broadly defined by Europe, but giving expression to perceptions of the particular local causes of disease through the impact of climate, vegetation and physical topography.[28] In an age still influenced by the views of Montesquieu, Hume and Falconer about the effects of climate and geography on human society and nature, this interest in medical topography served to strengthen the concept of disease as being environmentally determined, a paradigm (in the Kuhnian sense) that especially fitted the understanding of the exceptional dangers of tropical climates.

Finally, even aesthetic taste had implications for changing medical representations of the tropics. In their descriptions medical writers of the late eighteenth and early nineteenth century frequently deployed the literary convention of calling tropical landscapes 'picturesque', even 'sublime'. The islands of the West Indies and the coast of West

Africa were singled out for the beauty of their hills or the 'wild exuberance' of their vegetation.[29] But this appreciation of the 'sublime' and the 'picturesque', rather than contradicting the image of the perilous tropics, served rather to reinforce it, for behind every enticing vista lurked a lethal miasma. The tropics were treacherous as well as dangerous, their beauty a deadly deception. Alexander Bryson, a naval surgeon and leading medical statistician, made precisely this point about Fernando Po in the 1840s. 'The island, taken as a whole, is perhaps one of the most beautiful on the face of the earth', he wrote enthusiastically. It had few rivals anywhere in its 'sublimity and grandeur', and yet, as the medical statistics showed, there was not 'any spot in the whole world more detrimental to health'.[30]

As scientific experts as well as medical practitioners, doctors and surgeons not only reported on the tropics – in some senses they also invented them, investing the distinctiveness of their flora and fauna, their climates, soils and vegetation, with a scientific precision and a pathological potency that marked them out from milder, more temperate lands. Despite the tendency in the new tropical medicine of the late nineteenth century to eschew climate and topography in favour of bacilli and protozoa, there remained a sense in which the physical and social peculiarities of Africa, Asia and the central regions of the Americas, continued to inform the medical discourse and praxis.

Chronologies and Connections

It is also important to try to establish a chronology for our subject, one which acknowledges the impact of debates and discoveries in medicine in Europe, but also registers those events which, while tracing their origins or motive force to Europe, were yet enacted far from its shores – the subjugation of the Americas, the trans-Atlantic slave trade, the successive establishment of Portuguese, Dutch and British power in the East. Such a chronology, important to our subject in itself, may also allow us to question many of the Eurocentric assumptions of medical history, which has been slow to recognize the contributions that Western medicine in the tropics made to the development of metropolitan medical science – for instance, through the adoption of new drugs from America and Asia, through such practices as smallpox inoculation, or the early introduction of Chinese practices of acupuncture and moxibustion. One could go further and argue that European medicine was only able fully to universalize itself – to show itself more than the local lore of white men and Western Europe – through its protracted trials, encounters and appropriations overseas.

For much of our period maritime trade and sea power was the key to European involvement, and much of the medicine of the period duly reflected this maritime dependency – in the nature of the diseases observed and prescribed for, in the places where medicine was practised, and in the people who were its patients and practitioners.[31] In some senses, then, this medicine was doubly peripheral: it was distant from Europe but also stood on the outer margins of the vast continents of Africa and Asia. Of particular importance to the history of Europe's medicine overseas was, in consequence, that moment of transition, when Europe moved from sea to land, from maritime trade to territorial empire, and greatly increased the degree of its involvement with other peoples and places. Exceptionally, in parts of the Americas, this moment came early on in the history of European (and specifically Iberian) expansionism, with consequences which have barely begun to be considered,[32] while in India, Southeast Asia and much of Africa it was slower to arrive, coming only during the eighteenth or nineteenth centuries.

One of our needs (and opportunities) is to see Europe's medical ventures overseas as more than just a series of independent national narratives; to view them instead in a comparative, transnational perspective.[33] We already have begun to acquire, if often in antiquarian fashion, the histories of European medicine in individual territories around the globe and of the ties of dependence between them and Europe. But we have had little sense of the degree to which medical networks transcended national and imperial divisions, or how medical knowledge was passed on, over time as well as across space, from one European power to another. Is this a history of accumulating knowledge and unfolding common purposes or of multiple breaks and disjunctures? Was there, for instance, much con-tinuity of medical ideas and practices between the Portuguese, Dutch and English physicians in the East Indies between 1500 and 1750 or between the English and French in West Africa and the Caribbean in the eighteenth and nineteenth centuries?

As several essays in this volume suggest, there were, in fact, a number of lateral connections between tropical and colonial territories, as well as between them and the metropolis. The works of d'Orta and Bontius were clearly widely known outside their home countries and in editions other than those of their original place and language. As late as the nineteenth century British physicians in India were turning to d'Orta for evidence of the earlier history of cholera and its treatment,[34] while Bontius' study of the medical drugs and plants of the East Indies, first published in Amsterdam in 1658, though not translated into English until 1769, became widely known to physicians elsewhere in the tropical world, notably in the English and French West Indies in the eighteenth century, where he was cited as an authority on dysentery, tetanus and the effects of tropical climates in general.[35] James Lind's *Essay on Diseases Incidental to Europeans in Hot Climates,* first published in 1768, similarly had a wide and enduring reputation. Even at a time of bitter Anglo-French rivalry, a French translation was published in Paris in 1785 and was cited with approval by Thévenot in his discussion of disease in West Africa in 1840.[36] A remarkably large number of works of this genre were translated into other European languages – there was, somewhat surprisingly, a German edition of John Hunter's 1788 *Observations on the Diseases of the Army in Jamaica* published in Leipzig only four years later.[37]

Physicians themselves clearly made connections between their respective areas – in particular, in the late eighteenth century, between those two poles of European commercial and maritime rivalry, the East and West Indies. But it also needs to be stressed (as several contributors to this volume remind us) that the notion of 'warm climates' extended the basis of comparison well beyond the tropics as such – to the Maghreb and the southern shores of Europe itself. George Cleghorn's *Observations on the Epidemical Diseases in Minorca from the Year 1744 to 1749* was, significantly, often cited in the late eighteenth- and early nineteenth-century tropical literature, especially for its account of malarial fever, as indeed were the works of Thomas Sydenham.[38] The connection was often not the tropics as geographically defined but the nature and treatment appropriate to specific diseases, such as malaria, common to several parts of the globe, or, as perhaps in the case of Hunter's book on Jamaica, of wider relevance to military health and hygiene.

Another way of approaching the question of transnational linkages would be to ask what the role was of medical institutions in Europe in the dissemination of medical ideas and practices. Medical schools and universities like those in Leiden, Edinburgh and Paris in the eighteenth and nineteenth centuries provided a medical training that transcended state boundaries and, in the spirit of the Enlightenment, helped foster a common medical culture. Leiden and Edinburgh, were for example, the main source of medical training for doctors in the English-speaking West Indies in the eighteenth century.[39] Moreover, the doctors and surgeons to be found in the service of the Dutch East India Company in the seventeenth and eighteenth centuries included Swedes and

Germans as well as Dutchmen, just as the Brazilian doctors of the Bahian 'Tropicalista' School had connections by birth, training or medical orientation with Britain, Germany and France.[40]

But again, metropolitan origins and links do not supply the whole story. Medical practitioners were profoundly influenced by the local conditions they encountered – whether in Java or Jamaica, Senegal or Surinam. They were always more than mere messengers for metropolitan medicine. Sometimes it was the challenge of a new disease environment that caused doctors to question, innovate, or look to indigenous practice for guidance (though as in sixteenth-century Goa, such moments of mutual observation and interaction might be singularly shortlived). At times there was a fruitful interaction with indigenous medicine, even in areas where one might have expected the colonialists to have been most antipathetic to indigenous society and culture, as in Mexico. Indeed, it has been claimed that 'a large proportion of the European medical therapies of the sixteenth, seventeenth, and eighteenth, and part of the nineteenth centuries was based on new medicines imported from America'.[41] Among these were cinchona, ipecacuanha, jalap and balsam[42] – drugs also extensively used in the West Indies and India by the late eighteenth and early nineteenth centuries. Institutions, too, might flourish in overseas territories more readily than they did in Europe itself. For instance, in Portguese Goa, in Spanish Mexico and the Dutch East Indies hospitals often assumed greater importance (and indeed, to judge by the experience of Goa, were often on a more lavish scale and attracted greater state support) than in Europe itself.[43] All this suggests that for a variety of reasons (some of them explored and illustrated in this volume) tropical medicine was often the result of a 'synergetic relationship between core and periphery' rather than, as has often been assumed in the past, a simple transference or imposition of European ideas and techiques.[44]

We also need to know more about the professional channels through which medical ideas and practices related to the tropics were generated and disseminated – the army, the navy, colonial governments, municipal bodies, and religious organizations – and what medical schools and learned societies contributed to the networking of medical knowledge. Several essays in this collection attest to the importance of locally published works, especially medical journals like the *Indian Medical Gazette,* the *Gazeta Medica da Bahia,* or the publications of the Pasteur Institutes, in the development of distinctive local schools of medical thought and research. The scale and nature of this earlier knowledge may in time do much to question the originality of the tropical medicine of the late nineteenth century, or at least to explain how a new specialty, once it had come into being, was able to make such rapid progress around the globe. The groundwork had arguably already been done: the networks were in place. Indeed, Manson and Ross, rather than being lone pioneers, are perhaps now better understood as prime exponents of how effectively these solid overseas foundations could be built upon to capture medicine in the metropolis.

Clearly, the approaches adopted in these essays do not exhaust the rich possibilities opened up by the new and growing interest in pre-Mansonian tropical medicine. For instance, medical source materials can also, despite their biases and errors, provide unique insights into indigenous beliefs and practices from the earliest stages of a European presence, and yield otherwise elusive information about the nature and incidence of particular diseases and general levels of mortality. But this is a potentially rich research field – alike for historians, demographers, anthropologists and epidemiologists. Our hope here is simply to have brought together some illustrations of how this long period of observation, interaction and assimilation can begin to be opened up for further investigation and analysis.

Notes

1. A. J. Duggan, 'Medicine and health in the tropics: A brief history of Britain's role', *Transactions of the Royal Society of Tropical Medicine and Hygiene,* lxxv (1981), 5.
2. H. H. Scott, *A History of Tropical Medicine* (London: Arnold, 1939), I, v, 3; II, 1073–4; cf. P. H. Manson-Bahr and A. Alcock, *The Life and Work of Sir Patrick Manson* (London: Cassell, 1927), 208–9.
3. J. Farley, *Bilharzia: A History of Imperial Tropical Medicine* (Cambridge: Cambridge University Press, 1991), 13–23. Worboys lists eight schools or departments of tropical medicine established in Europe and North America between 1899 and 1913, in addition to two chairs of tropical medicine: M. Worboys, 'Tropical diseases', in W. F. Bynum and R. Porter (eds), *Companion Encyclopedia of the History of Medicine* (London: Routledge, 1993), I, 520. One could add other institutions, both in Europe and overseas, such as the Calcutta School of Tropical Medicine, opened in 1920, and various associations such as the Society of Tropical Medicine and Hygiene in Britain (of which Manson was the first President) founded in 1907, and its Dutch equivalent, the Nederlandsche Vereeniging voor Tropische Geneeskunde, launched the same year. For the emergence of tropical medicine in The Netherlands, see G. M. van Heteren, 'The course in tropical medicine at Amsterdam: "A case of monopolization"?', in G. M. van Heteren, A. de Knecht-van Eekelen

and M. J. D. Poulison (eds), *Dutch Medicine in the Malay Archipelago, 1816–1942* (Amsterdam: Rodopi, 1989), 35–55.

4. Worboys, *op. cit.* (note 3), 518; *idem,* 'The emergence of tropical medicine: A study in the establishment of a scientific specialty', in G. Lemaine *et al.* (eds), *Perspectives on the Emergence of Scientific Disciplines* (The Hague: Mouton, 1976), 75–98.
5. For Laveran's importance, see E. Sergent, 'La médecine française en Algérie', *Archives de l'Institut Pasteur d'Algérie,* xxxii (1954), 283. Of Koch, Duggan observed, 'only after [his] proof of the germ theory of disease in 1874 were tropical diseases approached in a scientific way': *op. cit.* (note 1), 5; and for Pasteur and the innovative role of the Pasteur Institutes in tropical medicine, see A. M. Moulin in this volume and 'Patriarchal science: The network of the overseas Pasteur Institutes', in P. Petitjean, C. Jame and A. M. Moulin (eds), *Science and Empires: Historical Studies about Scientific Development and European Expansion* (Dordrecht: Kluwer, 1992), 307–22; also A. Marcovich, 'French colonial medicine and colonial rule: Algeria and Indochina', in Roy MacLeod and Milton Lewis (eds), *Disease, Medicine and Empire: Perspectives on Western Medicine and the Experience of European Expansion* (London: Routledge, 1988), 109–14. For Finlay and Reed, see C. M. Wilson, *Ambassadors in White: The Story of American Tropical Medicine* (Port Washington: Kennikat Press, 1972), Chs 4 and 5.
6. Some at least of Manson's claims for the importance of tropical medicine were voiced by W. C. Maclean as the retiring Professor of Military and Clinical Medicine at Netley in 1886: W. C. Maclean, *Diseases of Tropical Climates* (London: Mamillan, 1886), 1–16. For the somewhat sceptical response of the Indian medical establishment to Manson and the 'boom in tropical medicine', see K. McLeod's 'London Letter', *Indian Medical Gazette,* June 1899, 215, and December 1899, 456. See also Worboys, 'The emergence of tropical medicine' (note 4), 87 and M. Harrison in this volume.
7. A. Balfour, 'Some British and American pioneers in tropical medicine and hygiene', *Translations of the Royal Society of Tropical Medicine and Hygiene,* xix (1925), 189–229. Cf. L. Jan Bruce-Chwatt, 'The rise of tropical medicine: Milestones of discovery and application', in C. G. Bernhard, E. Crawford and P. Sorbom (eds), *Science, Technology and Society in the Time of Alfred Nobel* (Oxford:Perganmon Press, 1982), 167: 'Few if any chapters of medical history have seen such an explosive rise and development as that of tropical medicine, which was born and grew during the years 1830–1900'.
8. H. W. Mulligan, 'Tropical medicine and research in British territories overseas', *Transactions of the Royal Society of Tropical Medicine and Hygiene,* lxxv (1981), 9.
9. E. Chernin, 'Patrick Manson (1844–1922) and the transmission of filariasis', *American Journal of Tropical Medicine and Hygiene,* xxvi

(1977), 1065.

10. P. Manson, 'The necessity for special education in tropical medicine', *Lancet,* ii, (1897), 842–5.
11. P. Manson, *Tropical Diseases: A Manual of the Diseases of Warm Climates* (London: Cassell, 1898); Duggan, *op. cit.* (note 1), 5.
12. S. May, 'Economic interest in tropical medicine', *American Journal of Tropical Medicine and Hygiene,* iii (1954), 413–15; B. Maegraith, 'Tropical medicine: What it is not, what it is', *Bulletin of the New York Academy of Medicine,* xlviii (1972), 1210–14; D. Bradley, 'Tropical medicine', in J. N. Walton *et al.* (eds), *The Oxford Companion to Medicine* (Oxford: Oxford University Press, 1986), II, 1393–9. 'By tropical medicine was actually meant colonial medicine, i.e., that branch of medicine dealing with diseases that for the most part were not tropical *per se* but were prevalent in tropical colonies and which were therefore of intense practical interest to colonial powers': E. H. Ackerknecht, *History and Geography of the Most Important Diseases* (New York: Hafner, 1965), 4.
13. Roy MacLeod observes that 'from the late 1870s, this tropical medicine – its ideology European, its instrument the microscope, its epistemology the germ theory of disease – served the interests of dominant economic groups and obscured the relationship of disease to social structure': 'Introduction' to MacLeod & Lewis (eds), *op. cit.* (note 5), 7. See also the other essays in MacLeod & Lewis, and David Arnold (ed.), *Imperial Medicine and Indigenous Societies* (Manchester: Manchester University Press, 1988); Farley, *op. cit.* (note 3), Ch. 2; Worboys, *op. cit.* (note 3), and his essay in this volume.
14. Notably, P. D. Curtin, 'The white man's grave: Image and reality', *Journal of British Studies,* i (1961), 94–110; *The Image of Africa: British Ideas and Action, 1780–1850* (Madison: University of Wisconsin Press, 1964); *idem, Death by Migration: Europe's Encounter with the Tropical World in the Nineteenth Century* (Cambridge: Cambridge University Press1989).
15. For example, K. D. Patterson and G. W. Hartwig (eds), *Disease in African History* (Durham, N.C.: Duke University Press, 1978); MacLeod & Lewis (eds), *op. cit.* (note 5), Arnold (ed.), *op. cit.* (note 13).
16. Modern tropical medicine has similarly never been satisfied with a purely geographical definition. Manson, *op. cit.* (note 11), xi, admitted that the term tropical diseases was 'more convenient than accurate', and continued 'If by "tropical diseases" be meant diseases peculiar to, and confined to, the tropics, then half a dozen pages might have sufficed for their description...' Cf. Scott, *op. cit.* (note 2), I, vi.
17. J. M. Cohen (ed.), *The Four Voyages of Christopher Columbus* (London: Hutchinson, 1969), 64, 66, 70, 85; J. H. Elliott, *The Old World and the New, 1492–1650* (Cambridge: Cambridge University Press, 1970).

18. Quoted in J. Prest, *The Garden of Eden: The Botanical Garden and the Re-Creation of Paradise* (New Haven: Yale University Press, 1981), 34.
19. W. Bosman, *A New and Accurate Description of the Coast of Guinea* (London: Knapton and Midwinter, 1705), 245; J. Hunter, *Observations on the Disease of the Army in Jamaica* (London: Nicol, 1788), 6–7; B. Moseley, *A Treatise on Tropical Diseases, on Military Operations, and on Climate of the West-Indies,* 2nd edn, (London: Cadell, 1789), 10–12, 36.
20. R. Towne, *A Treatise of the Disease Most Frequent in the West-Indies* (London: Clarke, 1726), 1–2, 11–12; P. Desportes, *Historie des Maladies de S. Domingue* (Paris: Lejay, 1770), I, 17–19; T. Dancer, *The Medical Assistant or Jamaica Practice of Physic Designed Chiefly for the Use of Families and Plantations* (Kingston, Jamaica: Aikman, 1801), iii; J. Annesley, *Researches into the Causes, Nature and Treatment of the Most Prevalent Disease of India, and of Warm Climates Generally* (London: Longman, 1828), I, xi, 7. On miasmatic theory in general, see Caroline Hannaway, 'Environment and miasma', in W. F. Bynum and R. Porter (eds), *Companion Encyclopedia of the History of Medicine,* I, 292–308.
21. W. Hillary, *Observations on the Changes of the Air and the Concomitant Epidemical Diseases in the Island of Barbadoes,* 2nd edn, (London: Hawes, Clarke and Collins, 1766), i; cf. Towne, *op. cit.* (note 20), 1; Moseley, *op. cit.* (note 19), xv. See also M. A. Osborne's essay in this volume for the 'resurrection' of Hippocrates in early nineteenth-century France.
22. Hillary, *op. cit.* (note 21), 140, 304, 339.
23. These developments and their significance are discussed more fully here by Kiple and Ornelas.
24. For example, R. Jackson, *A Treatise on the Fevers of Jamaica* (London: Murray, 1791), iii–v.
25. In particular, see Dancer, *op. cit.* (note 20), Hillary, *op. cit.* (note 21), W. F. Daniell, *Sketches of the Medical Topography and Native Diseases of the Gulf of Guinea, Western Africa* (London: Highley, 1849); W. Twining, *Clinical Illustrations of the More Important Diseases of Bengal,* 2nd edn, (Calcutta: Mission Press, 1835), II, 417–38. The importance of this dimension of early tropical medicine has been most effectively shown for the West Indies by R. B. Sheridan, *Doctors and Slaves: A Medical and Demographic History of Slavery in the British West Indies, 1680–1834* (Cambridge: Cambridge University Press, 1985).
26. H. Marshall, *Notes on the Medical Topography of the Interior of Ceylon* (London: Burgess and Hill, 1821), vi; Annesley, *op. cit.* (note 20). For the earlier narratives, see Hillary, *op. cit.* (note 21); Desportes, *op. cit.* (note 20), I.
27. D. G. Carlson, *African Fever: A Study of British Science, Technology and Politics in West Africa, 1787–1864* (Canton MA: Science History

Publications, 1984), Ch. 5; Curtin's essay below.

28. See Daniell, *op. cit.* (note 25), J. R. Martin, *Notes on the Medical Topography of Calcutta* (Calcutta: Huttmann, 1837); and, more generally, J. C. Riley, *The Eighteenth-Century Campaign to Avoid Disease* (Basingstoke: Macmillan, 1987), Ch. 2.
29. Daniell, *op. cit.* (note 25), 9–10, 49; C. Chisholm, *An Essay on the Malignant Pestilential Fever Introduced into the West Indian Islands from Boullam, on the Coast of Guinea* (London: Dilly, 1795), 2–6; C. J. Glacken, *Traces on the Rhodian Shore: Nature and Culture in Western Thought from Ancient Times to the End of the Eighteenth Century* (Berkeley: University of California Press, 1967), Ch. 12.
30. A. Bryson, *Report on the Climate and Principal Diseases of the African Station* (London: Clowes, 1847), 21–2; cf. Hunter, *op. cit.* (note 19). Although the term 'picturesque' was widely used by European artists and travellers in India at the time, I have seen no such usage in the extensive medical writing.
31. J. Watt, 'Medical aspects of the long voyages of exploration', in M. G. Marques and J. Cule (eds), *The Great Maritime Discoveries and World Health* (Lisbon: Escola Nacional de Saúde Pública, 1991), 19–38; R. B. Sheridan, 'The Guinea surgeons on the Middle Passage: The provision of medical services in the British slave trade', *International Journal of African Historical Studies,* xiv (1981), 601–25.
32. See J. Peard's essay below; also S. A. Alchon, *Native Society and Disease in Colonial Ecuador* (Cambridge: Cambridge University Press, 1991).
33. Curtin's *Death by Migration* is a pioneering work in this respect.
34. For d'Orta, see M. N. Pearson's essay below; J. MacPherson, *Annals of Cholera from the Earliest Periods to the Year 1817* (London: Ranken, 1872), 85–7.
35. For Bontius, see P. Boomgaard in this volume; Towne, *op. cit.* (note 20), 3; Hillary, *op. cit.* (note 21), 219; Desportes, *op. cit.* (note 20), I, 18; Moseley, *op. cit.* (note 19), 19, 314–17.
36. J.-P.-F. Thévenot, *Traité des Maladies des Européens dans les Pays Chaud et Spécialement au Sénégal* (Paris: Baillière, 1840), 375.
37. For this and other titles, see A. Hirsch, *Handbuch der Historisch-Geographischen Pathologie,* lst edn (Stuttgart: Enke, 1860), 3 vols; English translation, *Handbook of Geographical and Historical Pathology* (London: New Sydenham Society, 1883–6). Hirsch lists a remarkable number of French and English works on tropical medicine as well as German translations and original texts.
38. G. Cleghorn, *Observations on the Epidemical Diseases in Minorca from the Year 1744 to 1749* (London: Wilson, 1751).
39. Sheridan, *op. cit.* (note 25), 56.
40. See the essays by Boomgaard and Peard below. For discussion of the status of doctors in British overseas territories and services, see D. M. Haynes' essay, in this volume.

41. C. S. Kidwell, 'Aztec and European medicine in the New World, 1521–1600', in L. Romanucci-Ross, D. A. Moerman and L. R. Tancredi (eds), *The Anthropology of Medicine: From Culture to Method* (New York: Praeger, 1983), 20–31; G. Schendel, *Medicine in Mexico: From Aztec Herbs to Betatrons* (Austin: University of Texas Press, 1968), 86–8.
42. F. Guerra, 'Medical colonization of the New World', *Medical History*, vii (1963), 153.
43. As well as Pearson and Boomgaard in this volume, see A. J. R. Russell-Wood, *Fidalgos and Philanthropists: The Santa Casa da Misericordia of Bahia, 1550–1755* (London: Macmillan, 1968), and Guenter Risse, 'The encounter between Aztec and Spanish medical cultures: Hospitals in sixteenth-century Spain', paper presented to the Wellcome Symposium on 'Tropical Medicine Before Manson', London, 25 March, 1993.
44. M. A. Osborne, 'The medicine of the hot countries, philology and European settlement in Algeria, 1830–1870', paper presented at the Davis Center, Princeton University, 19 April, 1991; Harrison, 'Social construction'.

1

First Contacts between Indian and European Medical Systems: Goa in the Sixteenth Century

M. N. Pearson

Until the sixteenth century medical knowledge in Europe, in the Muslim world and in India seems to have been relatively evenly spread. No area had any decisive advantage, although in different specialties different areas were ahead. Most obviously, healers in India had been practising 'tropical medicine' long before Europeans reified the concept and appropriated it to describe their own halting attempts to deal with 'warm climate' diseases. There was a considerable degree of interaction between the traditional systems of these three areas, yet there was also a recognition that some illnesses were geographically specific. Some Indian illnesses, for example, were seen by foreigners as 'different'. This interaction, and also the notion of difference, was seen in India in the sixteenth century, especially in the Portuguese capital of Goa. Indeed, these themes are plain to see in the career and writing of sixteenth-century Goa's greatest savant, the New Christian Garcia d'Orta and a study of his work will conclude this essay.

Plague, smallpox and syphilis were three of the most threatening diseases in Europe at the time. In Portugal in the period of the discoveries, that is in the fifteenth and sixteenth centuries, all three of these diseases were found in abundance. There were several major plague epidemics in the sixteenth century. Plague had originated in Asia, but we cannot tell whether these particular epidemics came from within Europe, or from India, or indeed whether the plague went from Portugal to India. It is possible that both areas had indigenous sources for this malady. In the major Portuguese plague epidemic of 1569–70, mortality in Lisbon in June 1569 was 50 to 60 a day, in July 300 to 400, and later up to 700. In this city of about 100,000 souls, some 50,000 died. Royal mortality in Portugal gives a good impression of general mortality, keeping in mind that royalty received the best care and had the best diets. D. Manuel, king from 1495 to 1521, had 13 children by three wives. Four of them predeceased him, and nine in all died before the age of 40. His successor, D. João III (1521–57), had ten children, whose average life span was 7.6 years: the oldest died at 22. Medical knowledge in Portugal, as in the rest of Europe, was incapable of dealing with these diseases.

As a result of the Muslim period of dominance in Portugal, which ended only in the late thirteenth century, Muslim authorities were widely used. Of the five books which in theory a druggist had to know before he could practise, four were of Muslim origin.[1] More generally, in Portugal, and indeed all of Europe, medicine was a blend of Latin, Arabic, Greek and Hebrew knowledge. In Portugal the most widely quoted authors were Hippocrates, Galen, Isaac and Ibn Sina (Avicenna). But these relatively scientific authorities blended easily into folk medicine, and belief in witches, astrology and sorcery. In other words, book-based medical practice co-existed with folk oral traditions.

One cure for diarrhoea was to rub the abdomen with egg whites, or with well-sifted goat dung, or a mixture of the two. In the thirteenth century Pedro Hispano, a very famous doctor and later to be Pope John XXI, said that a good cure-all was a little bag containing the eyes of a magpie, crab or wolf, worn around the neck. Badger powders were a very popular remedy:

> One began by inebriating a badger on a wine filtered through camphor and blended with a compound of gold, seed pearls, and coral. The animal then was decapitated, all of his blood drained, and his heart and liver removed. The mixture of the blood with the powders should be effected under a 'slow sun' or in the 'heat of a fire'.... Two ounces of paté resulting from pulverizing the heart, liver and even the skin and teeth of the badger completed the mixture. This compound, dissolved in wine or in water seasoned with vinegar, was given to the patient.[2]

We need more research on this interaction between formal and folk medicine, and must be careful not to ridicule folk practice. Andrew Wear claims in his recent edited collection of essays that 'the nineteenth- and twentieth-century values of the medical profession which in past history of medicine had been applied to earlier periods to condemn empirics, quacks, magical and religious practitioners have been discarded. In the process a much richer medical world has been uncovered.'[3]

Important advances occurred in European medicine, and especially surgery, during the Renaissance, but from the middle of the sixteenth century Portugal lost all chance of taking part in these changes. Medical education at the university in Lisbon in the early sixteenth century was traditional in the extreme. This university moved between Lisbon and Coímbra several times, until in 1537 Lisbon was definitively replaced by Coímbra. It seemed that this university was poised to take account of, and contribute to, medical and scientific advances in Renaissance Europe. Unfortunately, a relatively open intellectual atmosphere in Portugal early in the sixteenth century, and a Portuguese version of humanism, was stifled in the 1550s by the new Society of Jesus, and by the Inquisition, founded in 1536 and by mid-century dominant in the country. Its influence was especially detrimental at Coímbra, for many of the teachers there were New Christians.[4] As C. R. Boxer notes, until they were forced to convert in the late fifteenth century over 60 per cent of Portugal's doctors in Portugal had been Jews.[5] Persecution of them thus crippled medicine in Portugal. Indeed, in 1583 there was such a pronounced shortage of doctors in the kingdom that only one could be spared for India that year.[6]

By the late 1550s Hippocrates and Galen were firmly reestablished as the unquestioned and unquestionable authorities on all matters medical. This was doubly unfortunate for Portugal (and Spain) for the discoveries had opened up new horizons in all sorts of fields in the Iberian countries. In the case of medicine, Portuguese doctors and botanists soon found a host of new diseases and remedies. Garcia d'Orta and Cristovão da Costa listed these, but this was not considered to be acceptable knowledge in Portugal and the opportunity to pioneer in tropical medicine, and even contribute on the basis of this to new paradigms in European medicine, was never taken.

In most areas of disease and curing in early modern India there appears to have been no particular advantage in knowledge or skill on the part of the newly arrived Europeans. Rather it seems that, despite specific differences with regard to particular diseases, the situation overall was one of equality.[7] In certain areas, which could be loosely called 'tropical medicine,' Indian healers with their millennia of experience obviously knew more than did the Europeans.

We can now turn to the situation in the first large European settlement in India, the port of Goa which was conquered by Afonso Albuquerque for the Portuguese king in 1510, and was their main town and capital during the sixteenth century and later. The town's population in 1600 was about 75,000. Of these about 1,500 were

Portuguese or *mestiços* (ethnically mixed), 20,000 were Hindus, and some 50,000 were local Christians who had been converted during the sixteenth century. In the countryside the population was still predominantly Hindu.[8] Looked at from the late twentieth century, the prevalent diseases in sixteenth-century Goa make up a still familiar list. Late in the century a Dutch resident, Jan Hüygen van Linschoten, said the main ones were *mordexijn* (in other words cholera), the bloody flux (or dysentery), and fevers, especially malarial ones. The term 'fever'could cover a range of illnesses, which at this distance in time can hardly be specified. 'They have many continuall fevers, which are burning agues, and consume mens bodies with extreame heate, whereby within foure or five dayes they are eyther whole or dead,' wrote van Linschoten.[9] Pyrard de Laval, a visitor in the early seventeenth century, said burning fevers, presumably enteric fever (typhoid), and dysentery were common, as was venereal disease.

In Goa, syphilis, the disease which had devastated large parts of Europe after its probable introduction from America in the 1490s, was considered to be a Portuguese import. A local sixteenth-century Hindu work called it 'firangi roga', that is the 'European disease'.[10] Similarly, Pyrard claimed it was found only 'where the Portuguese are'.[11] It seems that a milder venereal disease was already widespread in India, so we can assume that he is referring here to the new, more virulent, American disease of syphilis. But van Linschoten in Goa in the 1580s must have been writing of the mild indigenous form when he noted:

> pockes and piles, with other secret diseases, they are in those countries verie common and not hidden or concealed, for they thinke it no shame, more then to have any other disease. They heale them with the roote China; there are some that have had them at the least three or foure times, and are not any thing at all shunned or disliked for the same, but dare both boast and bragge thereof. It is not anything perillous for the bodie...[12]

The question of cholera in sixteenth-century India is a controversial one. Some have claimed that cholera was first seen in the great pandemics that spread from India in the nineteenth century. But there is no doubt that what our sources describe in India in the sixteenth century was cholera. This is shown by the fact that all of the accounts stress rapid morbidity as a result of dehydration caused by acute watery diarrhoea: this must have been cholera, though it should be noted that the commonly described 'bloody flux' was not, for cholera does not produce internal bleeding. The point, presumably, is that there are various strains of the disease. One of these was epidemic in the sixteenth century, and possibly it was a variant of this that was so devastating three centuries later.

Cholera was a major killer in Goa. There were outbreaks in the town in 1543, 1563, 1567, 1570, 1580, 1588, 1610, 1635, 1639, 1670 and 1680. The first one was the worst; we are told that of those struck by it, only one in ten survived.[13] The Italian merchant Sassetti described it in Cochin in the 1580s:

> There is current here a certain disease which kills a person in just 24 hours and which is called *mordaxi,* which is a revulsion of the stomach and of the entire body which rejects itself; all the humours quit the body and the blood too, so that one dies; and it comes from eating much sweet fruit, much pork, many preserves, and from drinking much water; whence the poor stomachs, when they have suffered much, throw themselves on the ground. It is the accident which makes it known, that suddenly the patients lose the sense of touch in their external parts, so that they feel nothing if they are struck blows or pierced with a needle.[14]

The Venetian quasi-doctor Manucci later in the seventeenth century noted that *mort-de-chien,* or cholera, was the main killer, describing it as colic of the bowels with vomiting and laxity. The best cure, the usual one at this time, was to burn the heel of the patient with a red-hot iron until the heat was felt. In this way the pain was allayed and the discharge and vomiting stopped.[15]

Goa was generally considered to have a very high mortality rate. One estimate finds that no less than 25,000 Portuguese soldiers died in the Royal Hospital between 1604 and 1634; by repute 500 a year died from syphilis and 'the effects of profligacy'. As a proverb had it, 'Of the hundred who go to India [from Portugal], not even one returns.'[16] Many in fact never even made it to India, such was the mortality on the voyage out from Lisbon. Vasco da Gama on his first voyage lost over half his crew to scurvy. Duncan shows that between 1497 and 1590 some 171,000 people left Lisbon for the east, and about 17,000 of these were lost to disease or shipwreck.[17] When the great ships from Portugal arrived each year in Goa they brought with them many newcomers with bad ulcers, the result of scurvy.[18] Accounts of the state of health on board the great carracks arriving in Goa from Lisbon are harrowing in the extreme.[19] A contemporary list shows that in the period 1629–34 5,228 people left Portugal for India, but only 2,495 completed the voyage – though to be sure some would have deserted, and two ships of the 17 that left Portugal in this period were lost at sea.[20] As one other indication of mortality, which reflects the mortality of the royal family at home, of 50 governors of Portuguese India up to 1656, 22 died during their term of office or on their way home.

Several travellers speculated on the reasons for Goa's unhealthiness. Manucci and others put forward the notion that India was healthy for men over the age of 40, but not for younger men. As Dr John Fryer put it, 'For to the Lustier and Fresher, and oftentimes the Temperatest, the Clime more unkind; but to Old Men and Women it seems to be more suitable.'[21] Medical practice at the time also contributed to high mortality, a point we will return to shortly. One problem was Goa's porous soil, so that sewage sank into drinking wells, and thus faecal-borne disease was spread. There seems also to have been an increase in the incidence of malaria due to stagnant waters lying around. Manucci left a vivid picture of illness and mortality in Goa. In his view, the unwholesome air in Goa was a problem. Also there was an island nearby which was a real graveyard:

> The reason is that it is full of courtesans, Mahomedan and heathen, who bear on them the unhappy poison by which they take the life of so many wretched men, after they have like leeches sucked from them every penny in their purse. It is, above all, the soldiers newly arrived from Portugal who succumb to this sad fate. Having exhausted both their bodily strength and their scantily-stored purses in the infamous dens allowed to exist there, misery and feebleness overtake them so completely that they are forced to enter the hospital. That is a place from which they hardly ever come forth alive, the number of men dying there being astonishing, every day five to 25 dead bodies being carried out, sometimes more, sometimes less, a fact that I have myself observed several times. By this means that island becomes the cemetery of all those newly arrived from Europe, and I honestly believe that at the end of the year not an eighth part survives of those who landed.[22]

Others, too, noted the effects of 'profligacy'. There was, of course, a real medical, as opposed to moral, basis for these comments, for the 'profligate' risked catching the new and more malignant venereal disease, syphilis, which the Portuguese had brought with them to India. Van Linschoten claimed that a fundamental cause of Portuguese ill health was that they

> use much company of women ... which often times costeth them both life and limme, for although men were of iron or steele, the unchaste life of a woman, with her unsatiable lustes were able to grinde him to powder, and sweep him away like dust, which costeth many a mans life.[23]

Whatever the reason, the health situation in Goa was so poor, and deteriorated so greatly during the seventeenth century, that in the eighteenth century the town was abandoned and the capital moved down river to the more healthy Panaji.

While some Indian diseases were well known from European experience others, such as cholera and enteric fever (typhoid), were unfamiliar to Portuguese doctors. The Italian merchant Sassetti noted in Malabar malaria, several sorts of apoplexy, and elephantiasis (or filaria). He also commented on different cures. Bleeding was seldom used, nor were such standards of European pharmacopoeia as rhubarb and aloe.[24] Many other commentators thought that Indian diseases were different, and should be treated by Indian methods. In the late seventeenth century an English doctor stressed the differences, and said gloomily that 'we are here, as Exotick Plants brought home to us, not agreeable to the Soil'.[25] But most European visitors were more sanguine and this in turn led to a very interesting eclectic mixture of Portuguese and Hindu medical systems.[26] David Arnold has noted how 'before 1800, Western medicine was far less domineering in its relationship with indigenous societies'. After this time, in the nineteenth century, the British rulers of India sometimes seemed to blame the Indians themselves for their ill health and high mortality. These were caused, it was claimed, by Indian culture and customs; the contribution of British colonialism was played down or ignored.[27] This seems to be a small illustration of the pronounced differences between the colonial impact of the two European powers. It is commonplace that an industrialized Britain had a much more overwhelming effect on India than did the Portuguese; indeed, I have several times made the case that the Portuguese had a very slight impact on most aspects of Indian life.[28] In the medical field, this smaller impact, even in their capital of Goa, and the essentially pre-modern nature of the Portuguese, meant that acculturation could flourish, and also that Indian mortality was seen as no different from Portuguese. Hence Hindu custom and medical practice were not blamed for disease and death.

The basic idea seems to have been that for certain diseases Indian doctors were much preferable to European ones. An extended contemporary Jesuit account noted how Hindu doctors

> come to the lands of the Portuguese, and they are examined by the Físico-Mór [the chief official Portuguese doctor], a man from Europe, whom I often heard stating that the said Brahmans called Panditas cure better than the European physicians who practise in India. I knew a friar of St Augustine, of the Portuguese nation, who taught medicine in Portugal, and lectured on it for sixteen years, who after coming to India treated some Portuguese patients, all of whom passed

> away; seeing this happening, the said priest called the Panditas and asked them how they went about curing their patients; they replied that the properties and the composition of the drugs were well taught in the books; however, this was not sufficient to heal the patient unless his complexion, and the ruling humour, and the connection with the local climate were first known, and that they ordered their remedies according to these principles. Knowing they were giving him a good reason, the Priest took some information from them in order to succeed in curing, and according to this and his science he later made some wonderful cures.[29]

The acceptance of this notion meant that for most of our period Indian medical practice was described, but usually without comment. Even though some of the 'cures' prevalent in India at this time seem today to be bizarre in the extreme, Europeans apparently found them different but not qualitatively better or worse than those they already knew. Van Linschoten even made a specific comparison of rival treatments of fevers:

> This sicknes is common and very daungerous, and hath no remedie for the Portingalles, but letting of blood: but the Indians and heathens do cure themselves with hearbes, Sanders, and other such like oyntments, wherewith they ease themselves. This sicknes consumeth many Portingalles every yeare.[30]

The related notions of a lack of qualitative difference, and the idea that Indian diseases were 'different', meant that even governors and clerics used Hindu healers because of their supposed better local knowledge. In 1548 an Indian Brahmin was practising in the Jesuit College of St Paul, and another *vaidya* (Hindu doctor, also sometimes called *pandit*) was doctor to Governor Barreto in 1574.[31] Governor Manuel de Sousa Coutinho (1588–91) and his wife were accused by the Inquisition of using Indian doctors, and dealing with Hindu sorcerers ['feiticeiros'].[32]

Portuguese racism sometimes tried to limit the prestige of these Hindu doctors. In 1572 the Governor decreed that Hindu teachers and doctors were not to go about on horseback or in palanquins. A first offence attracted a fine of ten cruzados, a second 20 cruzados and the loss of the offending horse or palanquin, and a third meant being sent to the galleys. However, the doctor who served the Governor's own household was exempt from this,[33] and in fact the prohibition soon lapsed. Van Linschoten noted in the 1580s that:

> There are in Goa many Heathen phisitions which observe their gravities with hats carried over them for the sunne, like the Portingales,

> which no other heathens doe, but onely Ambassadors, or some rich Marchants. These Heathen phisitions doe not onely cure there owne nations and countriemen but the Portingales also, for the Viceroy himselfe, the Archbishop, and all the Monkes and Friers doe put more trust in them then in their own countrimen, whereby they get great store of money, and are much honoured and esteemed.[34]

The Portuguese doctor Cristovão da Costa used to ask a local Brahmin doctor in Cochin about local cures; this doctor was popular among both Indians and Portuguese in the town.[35] In 1620 patients in the convent of Madre de Deus in Goa were treated by a *pandit,* and Portuguese soldiers wanting sick leave used letters from a *pandit.*[36]

The reverse of this sensible arrangement was that most governors brought their own doctors out with them from Lisbon as part of their vast retinues of relatives and hangers-on, all of them hoping to make a fortune in India during the three-year term of their patron. These newly arrived Portuguese doctors were nearly always rewarded by being made the chief doctor of the Royal Hospital, but several contemporaries noted that this was a prime cause of mortality, for they knew nothing of Indian diseases, and just as they began to acculturate they returned to Portugal with their gubernatorial patron.[37] In 1610 the king ordered that this practice cease and that the doctors and surgeons who went out with the viceroys not be allowed to practise in the Royal Hospital, 'because they have no experience of the region and its medical methods'. This order seems to have provoked a storm of complaints from Goa, and three years later it was lifted.[38] Another problem raised by these itinerant doctors, who usually returned to Portugal with their patron, was the resulting shortage of practitioners in Goa. A letter from Goa in 1644 complained of this, and noted despairingly that the present *fisico-mor* was a 'negro', in fact a Goan. The king was urged to take measures to make Portuguese doctors stay in Goa.[39]

There seems to be a contradiction here in Portuguese racial policies. As we have and will see, converted Jews, the 'New Christians', were greatly discriminated against, and Indian doctors were not allowed to practise in the Royal Hospital. Muslims generally were feared and disliked. As opposed to this, most Portuguese in India used Hindu doctors, and liked Hindu healing practice. It is inappropriate here to go into such a complex topic in any depth, but it may be suggested that the difference was between theory and practice, or perhaps normative as opposed to actual behaviour. Thus while Hindus and Jews, even New Christians, were to be discriminated against at an official or normative level, so that the former could not practise in the Royal Hospital, nor hold tax-farming contracts, in actuality they were still popular doctors, and held most of the contracts. Garcia d'Orta, of whom more later, seems to represent a paradigmatic figure in this respect. During his life he treated the Goan élite, from the governor on down. By contrast, after his death normative or official behaviour took over; he was accused of being a crypto-Jew and his bones were exhumed and ceremoniously burned.

Despite this discrimination, what we find overwhelmingly in Goa is a mixture of European and Hindu practice. As Arnold notes in the introduction to this book, tropical medicine appears more and more to have been the result of a synergistic relationship between core and periphery. Portuguese Goans seem to have had a quite *ad hoc* and experimental attitude to health, and tried different systems quite freely. An Augustinian friar with a very painful swelling in the testicles was cured by a poultice of stewed leaves applied by an old woman. A Hindu doctor was considered to know a perfect cure for scrofula, a swelling of the glands caused by tuberculosis. The Jesuits jealously guarded the recipe for their cordial stone, a bezoar stone with an amazing list of other ingredients added. It was used for heart problems, and was a good example of a mixture of Indian and European practice.[40] In the Portuguese settlement of Daman in 1673 a French visitor found a young Portuguese girl with fever, whose 'Indian physician, instead of letting her blood, had covered her head with pepper'. The European insisted on bleeding her with leeches, and perhaps surprisingly she recovered quickly. The use of pepper is obscure, but it may refer to the local practice of throwing pepper into the eyes of a sufferer. This was designed to gauge the severity of the malady. I assume that the point was that if patients did not react to the pepper they were given up for dead.[41] This incident points to a major divergence between European and Hindu medicine, which was the routine use of bleeding by Europeans.[42] Pyrard claimed Indians, that is Hindus, did not use bleeding at all.[43] There were clearly problems with this method of dealing with fevers, especially when it was used so often; patients in the Royal Hospital could be bled 30 or even 40 times.

Earlier European practice had combined bleeding with feeding up the patient. In the following description of medical practice in Goa's Royal Hospital from the 1640s we find that the Europeans had now decided that a much scantier diet was more appropriate. But we can also note that they were at least worried enough about the effects of bleeding to try to build up the patient, using a Hindu specific, after the bleeding was finished.

> I forgot to make a remark upon the frequent bleedings in reference to Europeans – namely, that in order to recover their colour and get themselves in perfect health, it is prescribed for them to drink for 12 days three glasses of *pissat de vache* [cow's urine], one in the morning, one at midday, and one in the evening; but, as this drink cannot but be very disagreeable, the convalescent swallows as little of it as possible, however much he may desire to recover his health. This remedy has been learnt from the idolaters of the country, and whether the convalescent makes use of it or not, he is not allowed to leave the hospital till the 12 days have expired during which he is supposed to partake of this drink.[44]

We have seen Europeans using Indian methods, and incorporating them into their medical practice. There was also some transfer of medical knowledge from India to Europe. John Ovington noted late in the seventeenth century:

> The general Ease and Cure, which the White Powder [?] in India gives to Feavers, makes that a very common and acceptable Receipt there; and it has, with very good Success, been administered in England, sent from thence by the Indian Physicians. And all their Medicines here are generally of the cooler sort, because of the Heats to which the Climate naturally inclines them.[45]

A decade or so earlier, Manuel Godinho said that some medicinal drugs were sent to dispensaries in Europe from India. They included miramulanos (a small medicinal fruit), asafoetida, spikenard and opium.[46] And despite the general European contempt for Asian surgery, India did make one important contribution here. The main activity in early plastic surgery was nose reconstruction, which in sixteenth-century Europe was done using a flap of skin. However, the church was opposed to this and the practice fell into disuse. The same method had been used in India for centuries. Information on this Indian practice reached Europe in the late eighteenth century, and revived European interest in rhinoplasty. On this foundation was built modern plastic surgery.[47]

What, however, of a reverse flow? Did Indians learn from the Portuguese? Certainly the great Portuguese healer and scholar Garcia d'Orta treated various rulers in the Deccan, especially the ruler of Ahmadnagar and his family, though he was often in competition with Muslim authorities at the court.[48] He claimed that the king 'taught me the names of illnesses and medicines in Arabic, and I taught him the same in Latin'. Hindu doctors often used Portuguese methods, 'But most of them not correctly.' Nevertheless, they had learned some things from European practice, just as d'Orta had from them.[49] At a meeting of the Portuguese Council of State in 1629 the ambassador of neighbouring Bijapur, who was meant to attend, excused himself because he was sick; he asked that the viceroy send him his *fisico-mor,* which the Portuguese agreed to do.[50] There is evidence from the seventeenth century of European surgeons being much in demand in India. This reflects the fact that Indian anatomy, and so surgery, was by this time well behind European knowledge, a point which Peter Boomgaard also notes in his essay in this book.

As for the universal European practice of bleeding, it seems to have been picked up by Hindu healers from the Portuguese quite early. D'Orta wrote acerbicly that 'they say there is bleeding [that is, that they practised it], and they never bled before we were in the land'.[51] By the later seventeenth century the method was more firmly established in areas where Europeans were numerous. In 1674–6 Dr Dellon was held in the prison of the Inquisition in Goa. Such was his despondency that he tired of life, and decided to end it, but wished to avoid a mortal sin by using someone else for the purpose. He feigned illness, and sure enough a doctor was introduced who prescribed five bleedings on five successive days. This remedy did indeed bring Dellon close to death, but more to the point the doctor was 'a Pundit, or Pagan Physician'.[52] Bleeding had never been used in Ayurvedic medicine, but in 1726 we are told that it was now very widely used by *pandits.* One used to bleed his patients up to 20 times. Such ferocious treatment was now less common in Europe, and indeed it appears that European patients were no longer prepared to tolerate this sort of treatment, for the French doctor added regretfully that this *pandit* could do this 'sans que les malades en murmurent, étant bien plus obeissans aux ordres de leur Medecin qu'on ne l'est en France'.[53]

The only area where the Portuguese were more advanced was in the matter of health care. Official bodies concerned themselves with the provision of medical facilities; apparently this was innovative for India. By late in the sixteenth century there were several hospitals in Goa. Among them was the Leper Hospital of St Lazarus, which had been founded in 1529.[54] The famous Royal Hospital of the Holy Spirit was Goa's main hospital. It had been founded by the conqueror of Goa, Afonso Albuquerque, to cater for Portuguese soldiers. Its main financing always came from the state, and in this it was truly new. At one time the revenues from the sale of the very valuable licensed voyage to China (Macao) were devoted to the hospital, and the king told the viceroy that if this did not suffice he was to write and say how much more was needed.[55] Admission was restricted to Portuguese soldiers and a few indigent Portuguese. It could cater for a very large total of 1,500 patients, and descriptions of it after it was expanded and rebuilt in the 1590s make it sound a most impressive structure indeed. Its staff included physicians, surgeons, apothecaries, barbers and bleeders, and Indian servants and slaves for the dirty work. No Indian doctors were allowed. Pyrard, who was a patient in 1608, has left an extended and glowing account of it. From his description the building looked like a grand palace. Even the beds were splendid, with mattresses and covers of silk or cotton. The meals were luxurious and ample, the plates, bowls and dishes of Chinese porcelain or even silver. On admission the patient had a hair-cut and wash, and was provided with bed-clothes.[56]

Why such a lavish establishment, apparently in advance of European hospitals at the time? The context is important. Such grandeur had a symbolically reassuring function. The hospital catered mostly for Portuguese soldiers, single men isolated in a precarious frontier society. In Portugal they could expect to be cared for by their families, but not in India. To maintain their loyalty (for many 'deserted' and sought greener pastures in neighbouring Indian states) it was important for the state to reassure them that they would be cared for if they were sick, and if they died, would die well. There is a similar divergence from European practice in the way that even the élite of Goa were happy to be cured in the hospital; in Europe at this time they would have seen a hospital as being only for the poor and indigent.

Given all this, why the appalling mortality in the hospital that we noted earlier? Among other reasons, the truly startling use of bleeding must have played a role, as also, no doubt, did the lack of Indian experience of the chief doctors. More basically, the underlying health problems of Goa, stagnant water and porous soils, could not be met by the existing state of medical knowledge. The causes of 'tropical diseases', such as cholera, dysentery and malaria, were not diagnosed until the the last century. Nevertheless, in the area of state involvement in public health and especially hospitals the Portuguese had an innovative role in India. Can we say the same about the greatest scholar of sixteenth-century Goa, the New Christian Garcia d'Orta (*c.*1500–68)? D'Orta was the first major naturalist to study the main medicinal plants and other therapeutic substances used in the East; he was also a doctor and historian of medicine, a pharmacist and a wide-ranging savant interested in history and anthropology. His famous work, *Colloquies on the Simples and Drugs of India,* was one of the first books (and one of the very few secular books) to be published in Goa in the sixteenth and seventeenth centuries. The rare first edition (only 24 copies are known) is dated 1563.[57] It is divided into 57 chapters, each of them in the form of a dialogue or colloquy. Each deals with one drug or simple. In each case he describes the drug, says where it grows, and comments on its therapeutic use. Most of the drugs are vegetable, but he also deals with ivory and diamonds. It is an excellent comprehensive and accurate empirical study of Indian materia medica and botany in general. It does not really discuss medicine as such, although he was a famous doctor in sixteenth-century Goa, serving as the physician of the Royal Hospital at the time of St Francis Xavier's stay in Goa in the early 1540s, and ministering to the Portuguese élite of the town and to local rulers.[58]

D'Orta's medical knowledge was not advanced. This can be seen from his description of cholera. Goa was hit by a major cholera epidemic in 1543: all classes and ages were struck by it in the winter, that is the monsoon period, of that year. The Portuguese doctors could do nothing, and of every 100 who were affected, only ten survived. Twelve, 15, even 20 victims were buried each day. The Governor, Martim Afonso de Sousa, even ordered an autopsy in a fruitless attempt to find the cause of the affliction.[59] D'Orta was the first European to publish a description of cholera in India. In the *Colloquies* he mentioned the Hindu and Arabic names for it, and compared what he saw in Goa with what he knew of Europe. He believed that there was a toxic humour which had to be expelled. It was caused by over-eating, or by too much sexual intercourse. He noted that the local *vaidyas* used rice with pepper and cardamom, cauterized the feet of the patient, tied up the patient's limbs and applied pepper to the eyes.[60] As to fevers, d'Orta followed European practice and treated fevers with bleeding and purging, and rich foods – the latter, as we noted, later lost favour in Goa. Thus we must not make too much of d'Orta's work. He seems to have been thoroughly grounded in early modern European practice of the first half of the sixteenth century. He learned of Muslim or Yunani medicine from its local practitioners, the *hakims,* and usually appreciated the abilities of the local *vaidyas* with whom he had contact, considering their cures as often superior to those he knew. However, he had no inkling of the vast and ancient body of Ayurvedic theory. The main influences on his medical thinking were the thoroughly predictable ones: Aristotle, Hippocrates, Galen and Ibn Sina. The basis of his work was, in essence, humoral pathology. His book goes into very elaborate detail as to whether various drugs were 'in the fourth, warm and dry', or 'in the second part of the third'.[61] D'Orta never went beyond this. He did correct and criticize his authorities on occasion, once, for example, writing 'Let not any text of any author deny what my own eyes have observed.... Frighten me not with Dioscorides or Galen, for I do not say but the truth and what I know.' [62] Nevertheless, he did not transcend them. It is especially revealing that he also quoted his contemporary Vesalius, but not on anatomy, in which he was the great paradigmatic innovator, but rather on a cure for syphilis.[63]

An important reason for this was the fact that d'Orta was a New Christian, and, apparently, a far from convinced convert. Born in *c.*1500, he studied at the Spanish universities of Salamanca and Alcalá de Henares, where his medical training consisted of memorizing Hippocrates, Galen and Ibn Sina. Subsequently d'Orta taught at Lisbon from 1526 until he left for India. It seems very likely that his departure for Goa in 1534, as the personal physician of the later Governor Martim Afonso de Sousa, was a result of increasing intolerance in Portugal. Two years after he left the Inquisition was set up in Lisbon, and was in full swing four years later. As a New Christian he was forced to step carefully, and no doubt he was also detrimentally affected by the mid-century attack on open inquiry which we mentioned above. As a result, the massive compilation that was the *Colloquies* was generally ignored in Portugal, though it was widely used in other parts of Europe in the later sixteenth century and subsequently, thanks to a Latin translation which went through five editions, the first one being published in 1567 in Antwerp. D'Orta himself suffered posthumously from this intolerance. He died in 1568, but in 1580 he was condemned as a Jew by the Inquisition, and his remains were dug up and burned at an *auto de fé*. A sister was burned by the Inquisition in Goa in the year after his death. Such intolerant bigotry symbolizes the stranglehold of the Counter Reformation as seen in the Inquisition on intellectual life in Portugal. While d'Orta certainly described many new (to Europeans) medicinal drugs and cures and diseases, and thus in a minor way contributed to undermine the authority of Hippocrates and Galen, it is incorrect to see him as representing a new paradigm for European medicine based on his Asian discoveries. Rather his contribution was to add to the store of European descriptive knowledge. [64]

Notes

Parts of this article are a much revised version of my 27th James Ford Bell lecture, presented to the Associates of the James Ford Bell Library, University of Minnesota, at the American Association of University Women's Club, Minneapolis, 3 May, 1989. The lecture was called 'Initial Contacts between European and Indian Medicine', and subsequently was published by the library. I am most grateful to Professor John Parker, the now retired Curator of this library, for inviting me to deliver this lecture. The present essay was greatly improved as a result of criticisms and comments at the conference from which this book comes. I must also thank Professor Donald Simpson, and my wife Denni, for helping to avoid at least some errors of medical fact. The present article could be read in tandem with my other venture into the history of medicine, 'The thin end of the wedge: Medical relativities as a paradigm of early modern Indian-European Relations', in *Modern Asian Studies,* 29 (1995), 141–70, which concentrates on the broader changes which occurred in the seventeenth century. Finally, much of my research into this subject was done, most appropriately, at the Xavier Centre of Historical Research in Goa. My thanks to its Director, Fr Teotonio de Souza, for his continued kindnesses over many years.

1. These were: *Pandectae Medicinae* by Matthaeus Sylvaticus; Mesua's *De Simplicibus; Antidotarium* by Nicolau Myrepso; *Liber Servitoris;* and the Fifth Book of the *Canon* of Ibn Sina. A. H. de Oliveira Marques, *Daily Life in Portugal in the Late Middle Ages* (Madison: University of Wisconsin Press, 1971), 151. A recent excellent introduction to Western European medicine in the fifteenth century is to be found in Roger French, 'Medicine in Western Europe during the fifteenth century', in Mario Gomes Marques and John Cule (eds), *The Great Maritime Discoveries and World Health* (Lisbon: Escola Nacional de Saúde Pública, 1991), 39–54.
2. Marques, *op. cit.* (note 1), 143–4.
3. Andrew Wear (ed.), *Medicine in Society: Historical Essays* (Cambridge: Cambridge University Press, 1992), Introduction, 2.
4. See P. D. Gaitonde, *Portuguese Pioneers in India: Spotlight on Medicine* (Bombay: Popular Prakashan, 1983), 75–81, for sketches of the careers of numerous doctors who left Portugal, often from Coímbra, as a result of religious distrust or even persecution, because they were Jews or 'New Christians' (that is, converted Jews).
5. C. R. Boxer, 'Some remarks on the social and professional status of physicians and surgeons in the Iberian World, 16th–18th centuries', *Revista de História* [São Paulo], 50 (1974), 199, 201.
6. King to Camara of Goa, 24 March, 1583, in J. H. da Cunha Rivara

(ed.), *Archivo Português Oriental* (Nova Goa: Imprensa Nacional, 1857–77, 6 vols), I, i, 95.

7. See Pearson 'The thin end of the wedge' for documentation.
8. For Goa in the sixteenth century, see M. N. Pearson, *The Portuguese in India* (Cambridge: Cambridge University Press, 1987), 81–115.
9. J. H. van Linschoten, *The Voyage of John Huyghen van Linschoten to the East Indies* (London: Hakluyt Society, 1885, 2 vols), I, 235–9. The quotation is from 236.
10. John M. de Figueiredo, 'Ayurvedic medicine in Goa according to European sources in the sixteenth and seventeenth centuries', *Bulletin of the History of Medicine,* 58 (1984) 227. This article provides a familiar sketch of some aspects of interaction, though the author's use of sources is occasionally careless (e.g., his footnote 14). An exhaustive search has failed to find any further publications by this author. For a recent and authoritative discussion of syphilis and its origins, see Ann G. Carmichael, 'Syphilis and the Columbian exchange: Was the new disease really new?' in Marques & Cule, *op. cit.* (note 1), 187–200.
11. François Pyrard de Laval, *The Voyage of François Pyrard of Laval to the East Indies* (London: Hakluyt Society, 1888), Vol. II, 11.
12. Linschoten, *op. cit.* (note 9), 239. See the following chapter by Boomgard for the 'China root' and its uses.
13. Alberto C. Germano da Silva Correia, *La Vieille-Goa,* (Bastorá: Tipografia Rangel, 1931) 268–307; see also his many other publications listed in the bibliography of this book. For the outbreak of 1567, see the contemporary Jesuit account in J. Wicki *et al.* (eds), *Documenta Indica,* (Rome: Jesuit Historical Institute, 1948 f., 16 vols to date) VII, 384, letter of Fr Gomes Vaz, 12 December, 1567. For the calamitous outbreak of 1570, see João Manuel Pacheco de Figueiredo, 'Goa dourada nos séculos XVI e XVII: O hospital dos pobres do padre Paulo Camerte, esboço de sua reconstituição histórica', *Studia,* 25 (1968), 136–40.
14. Quoted in John Correia-Afonso, 'On the fourth centenary of Filippo Sassetti (1540–1588): Scientific observations from Cochin', paper presented at the Fifth International Seminar on Indo-Portuguese History, Cochin, January 1989, and published in *Indica,* 26 (1989), 15–24. The quotation is from 19.
15. Niccolao Manucci, *Storia do Mogor, or Mogul India* (Calcutta: Editions Indian, 1966–67, 4 vols), II, 157. The word used for cholera in Goa was *mordexim* or variants thereof. Dalgado tells us that the word is local, deriving from the Konkani *modxi* or *morxi.* The French later converted it to *mort-de-chien.* See Sebastião Rodolfo Dalgado, *Glossário Luso-Asiático* (Coímbra: Imprensa da Universidade, 1919–21, 2 vols), s.v. 'mordexim', II, 69–71. According to H. G. Rawlinson the word came from the Marathi *modashi* through the Portuguese *mordexim.* See John Ovington, *A*

Voyage to Surat in the Year 1689, H. G. Rawlinson (ed.), (London, 1929), 204, footnote.

16. F. P. Mendes da Luz, 'Livro das Cidades', *Studia,* 6 (1960), fo. 8.
17. T. Bentley Duncan, 'Navigation between Portugal and Asia in the sixteenth and seventeenth centuries', in Cyriac K. Pullapilly *et al.* (eds), *Asia and the West: Encounters and Exchanges from the Age of Explorations: Essays in Honour of Donald F. Lach* (Notre Dame: University of Notre Dame, 1986), 3–25.
18. Pyrard de Laval, *op. cit.* (note 11), 11–14.
19. See Correia-Afonso, *op. cit.* (note 14), and Anthony Disney, 'The world of long-distance voyaging in the seventeenth century: The Lisbon-Goa fleet of 1629 as a case study', read at the International Symposium on Maritime History, Pondicherry, February 1989, and published in K. S. Mathew (ed.), *Studies in Maritime History* (Pondicherry: Pondicherry University, 1990), 143–58. See also A. J. R. Russell-Wood, 'Men under stress: The social environment of the Carreira da India, 1550–1750', *II Seminario Internacional de História Indo-Portuguesa, Actas* (Lisbon: Centro de Estudos de História e Cartografia Antiga, 1985), 19–35. For seventeenth-century mortality see da Cunha Rivara on board ship, *op. cit.* (note 6), I, ii, 197, Camara to King, letter of 1607, and J. H. da Cunha Rivara, 'A India no governo do ViceRei Conde de Villa Verde, 1693–1698', *O Chronista de Tissuary,* ii–iii (1868), 26: entry for 26 September, 1699. Philip Curtin has recently raised the matter of relocation costs in imperialism: evidence is lacking for the Portuguese, but I would strongly suggest that there was in fact a relocation cost in their empire, especially as even the actual relocation, that is the voyage out, was so expensive of life. Philip D. Curtin, *Disease and Imperialism before the Nineteenth Century* (Minneapolis: James Ford Bell Library, 1990) (Bell Lecture no. 28), and, more fully in *Death by Migration: Europe's Encounter with the Tropical World in the Nineteenth Century* (Cambridge: Cambridge University Press, 1989).
20. 'Livros das Monções do Reino', Historical Archives of Goa, Vol. 19B, f. 607, list of Barreto de Rezende.
21. Dr John Fryer, *A New Account of East India and Persia,* W. Crooke (ed.) (London: Hakluyt Society, 1909–15, 3 vols), I, 180; Manucci, *op. cit.* (note 15), II, 157.
22. *Ibid.,* III, 265.
23. Linschoten, *op. cit.* (note 9), I, 236–7.
24. Correia-Afonso, *op. cit.* (note 14), 19.
25. Fryer, *op. cit.* (note 21), I, 180.
26. I am aware that to write of 'Hindu' or 'Indian' medical practice is to ignore the pronounced regional differences evident at this time. Thus the important Portuguese commentator Cristovão da Costa differentiated between Brahmin, Canarin and Malabar treatments. See Jaime Walter (ed.), *Tratado das drogas e medicinas das India*

Orientais, por Christovão da Costa, (Lisbon: Junta de Investigações do Ultramar, 1964), 23, 28.

27. David Arnold, 'Introduction: Disease, medicine and empire', in David Arnold (ed.), *Imperial Medicine and Indigenous Societies* (Manchester: Manchester University Press, 1988), 11; *idem,* 'Occidental Therapeutics and Oriental Bodies: Bengal, 1800–1860', paper read at Subaltern Studies conference, Calcutta, December 1989.
28. See, for example, my *Portuguese in India,* (note 8), passim.
29. *Breve relação das escrituras dos gentios da India Oriental a dos seus costumes* (Lisbon: 1812), 52–3, quoted in de Figueiredo, *op. cit.* (note 10), 231. This and other descriptions of medical practice in sixteenth-century Goa raise an interesting general question. The generally accepted four stages of Western medical practice are: *library,* where practice was based on Galen and other authorities, and the healer had little contact with the patient; *bedside,* where observations were carried out; *hospital,* in other words huge wards of people, which developed in the nineteenth century; and *laboratory,* where doctors reveal the results of tests. What we find in Goa is a mixture of the first two of these typologies, or perhaps even the first three. Thanks to my colleague Dr Susan Hardy for introducing me to this matter.
30. Linschoten, *op. cit.* (note 9), I, 236.
31. J. M. Pacheco de Figueiredo, 'The practice of Indian medicine in Goa during the Portuguese rule, 1510–1699', *Luso-Brazilian Review,* 4 (1967), 52–3.
32. João Manuel Pacheco Figueiredo, 'Goa Pré-Portuguesa', *Studia,* 12 (1963), 139–259; 13–14 (1965), 105–225. The quotation is from 13–14, 163–4.
33. A. K. Priolkar, *The Goa Inquisition* (Bombay: 1961), 140.
34. Linschoten, *op. cit.* (note 9), I, 230.
35. Costa, *op. cit.* (note 26), 28. This experimental attitude was found early on in the Portuguese presence in the Indian Ocean. In 1505 some Portuguese engaged in taking Mombasa were hit by poisoned arrows. The Portuguese surgeon Mestre Fernando treated the wounds with wicks of pork fat, which soaked up the poison. He had learnt this technique from a Muslim healer. Fernão Lopes de Castanheda, *História do descobrimento e conquista da India pelos Portugueses* (Coímbra: Imprensa da Universidade, 1924–33, 9 vols, 3rd edn), II, 6.
36. de Figuereido, *op. cit.* (note 10), 231–2.
37. See Silva Correia, *op. cit.* (note 13), 275, and Pyrard, *op. cit.* (note 11), introduction, xii, and II, 14. For the career of one such *fisico-mor,* Dimas Bosque, who was attached to the viceroy D. Constantino de Bragança, 1558–61, see Jaime Walter, 'Dimas Bosque, fisico-mor da India a as sereias', *Studia,* 12 (1963), 261–71.
38. King to Viceroy, 23 January, 1610, in R. A. de Bulhão Pato (ed.), *Documentos remettidos da India, ou Livros das Monções* (Lisbon: Typografia de Academia Real das Sciencias, 1880–1935, 5 vols), I,

304, and King to Viceroy, 30 January, 1613, *ibid.*, II, 300.

39. Archivo Historico Ultramarino, Lisbon, caixa 16A, no. 160, letter of 7 September, 1644. My thanks to Timothy Coates of the University of Minnesota for this reference.
40. Ann Maria Amaro, 'Goa's famous cordial stone', *Review of Culture* [Macau], 7–8 (October 1988–March 1989), 82–103. Many thanks to Fr Charles Borges for this reference.
41. Priolkar, *op. cit.* (note 33), 14 of Dr Dellon's account.
42. On the use of bleeding in Portugal at this time, see, for copious and gory detail, Costa Santos, *Sobre barbeiros sangradores do hospital de Lisboa* (Porto: 1921).
43. Pyrard, *op. cit.* (note 11), II, 13.
44. Jean-Baptiste Tavernier, *Travels in India of Jean-Baptiste Tavernier*, trans. V. Ball and W. Crooke (New Delhi: Oriental Books Reprint Corporation, 1977, 2 vols), I, 160–1.
45. Ovington, *op. cit.* (note 15), 205.
46. John Correia-Afonso, (trans and ed.), *Intrepid Itinerant: Manuel Godinho and his Journey from India to Portugal in 1663* (Bombay: Oxford University Press, 1990), 70.
47. T. J. S. Patterson, 'The transmission of Indian surgical techniques to Europe at the end of the eighteenth century', in *Proceedings of the XXIII International Congress of the History of Medicine*, 2 vols (London: Wellcome Institute, 1974), I, 694–6. This paragraph is based on my article 'The thin end of the wedge'.
48. Clements Markham, *Colloquies on the Simples and Drugs of India by Garcia da Orta* (London: H. Sotheran, 1913), nos. 11, 13, 24, 36.
49. *Ibid.*, no. 36.
50. P. S.S. Pissurlencar (ed.), *Assentos do Conselho do Estado* (Bastorá: Tipografia Rangel, 1953–57, 5 vols), I, 237, meeting of 20 November, 1629.
51. D'Orta, *op. cit.* (note 48), no. 36.
52. Dellon in Priolkar, *op. cit.* (note 33), 42.
53. Luillier-Lagaudiers, *Nouveau voyage aux grandes Indes, avec une introduction pour le commerce des Indes Orientales, et la description de plusieurs isles, villes, & rivieres, l'histoire des plantes & des animaus qu'on y trouve; avec un traite des maladies particulieres aux pays orientaux, et dans la Route, et de leurs remedes* par Mr. D.L.F., Docteur en Medecine, qui a voyagé et sejourné dans les principales Villes des Indes Orientales (Rotterdam: 1726), 215. Portuguese records include copious detail on Hindu medical practice on the west coast of India in the sixteenth century, especially works by d'Orta, and Costa. These records will be used for a separate study on Hindu medicine in this period, but in terms of the present study the point is that the sources seem to show not superiority but acculturation and equality; the authors betray no feeling of contempt for Indian practice.
54. See C. R. Boxer, *Portuguese Society in the Tropics* (Madison: University

of Wisconsin Press, 1965), 24–6, and Silva Correia, *op. cit.* (note 13), 295–300. For another hospital founded in Goa in about 1550, called the 'Hospital dos pobres do Padre Paulo Camerte', see João Manuel Pacheco de Figueiredo, 'Goa dourada nos séculos XVI e XVII', 117–46.

55. King to Viceroy, 23 January, 1610, in Bulhão Pato, *op. cit.* (note 38), I, 303.
56. Pyrard, *op. cit.* (note 11), II, 2–17, provides the classic contemporary account of the Royal Hospital, while J. N. da Fonseca, *An Historical and Archaeological Account of the City of Goa* (Bombay: Thacker, 1878), 228–36, gives a good overview and references to documentary sources. The location of the Hospital can be worked out from the plan of Old Goa in his book; see also M. S. Commissariat (ed.) *Mandelslo's Travels in Western India, A.D. 1638–9* (Bombay: Oxford University Press, 1931), 70. I have in hand a separate study of the way the Portuguese tried to regulate medical practice in Goa, not only in their hospitals, but also in their attempts to license Hindu healers.
57. For d'Orta (and not Horta, da Orta, or Orta) see Garcia d'Orta, *Coloquios dos simplos, e drogas he cousas mediçinais de India* (Goa: Ioannes de Endem, 1563); Garcia da Orta, *Coloquios dos simples, e drogas he cousas mediçinais de India ...* Conde de Ficalho (ed.), (Lisbon: Imprensa Nacional, 1891–5, 2 vols); Markham, *op. cit.* (note 48), [a translation of Conde de Ficalho, Lisbon, 1891–5]. Especially important is C. R. Boxer, *Two Pioneers of Tropical Medicine: Garcia d'Orta and Nicolas Monardes* (London: Wellcome Institute, 1963). See also Conde de Ficalho, *Garcia da Orta e o seu tempo* (Lisbon: Imprensa Nacional, 1886); Luis de Pina, *Subsídios para a história da medicina portuguesa indiana do século XVII* (Porto: Araujo e Sobrinho, 1931); Luis Filipe de Sousa Barreto, 'Garcia da Orta e o dialogo civilizacional', in *Seminário internacional de história Indo-Portuguesa, Actas* (Lisbon: Centro de Estudos de História e Cartografia Antiga, 1985), 541–69, for a textual and semiotic study, and João Manuel Pacheco de Figueiredo, 'Coloquios dos simples de Garcia d'Orta, 1563–1963', *O Medico,* no. 602 (1963) (also published in *Boletim do Instituto Meneses Bragança,* 83 (1963), 161–86), for a useful summary, and also Gaitonde, *op. cit.* (note 4), 118–40. For more bibliography see Daya de Silva's excellent *The Portuguese in Asia: An Annotated Bibliography of Studies on Portuguese Colonial History in Asia, 1498–c.1800* (Zug: IDC, 1987), entry no. 2336, 252–3. There is even a journal named after him: *Garcia de Orta: Revista da Junta das Missões Geográficas e de Investigações do Ultramar,* Lisbon, 1952 – . This journal had an emphasis on scientific matters, and in 1963 in Vol. 9 no. 4, a special number commemorated the 400th anniversary of the publication of the *Coloquios.* The hagiography continues up to today. See Ivan A.

D'Cruz, 'Garcia da Orta in Goa: Pioneering tropical medicine', *British Medical Journal,* 303 (1991), 1593–4, and Fernando A. R. Nogueira, 'Garcia de Orta, physician and scientific researcher', in Marques & Cule, *op. cit.* (note 1), 251–64.

58. See Tomé Pires, *The Suma Oriental of Tomé Pires and the Book of Francisco Rodrigues* (ed. Armando Cortesão) (London: Hakluyt Society, 1944), 512–18, for an earlier and smaller account of Indian drugs; Jaime Walter, 'Simão Alvares e o seu rol das drogas da India', *Studia,* 10 (1962), 117–49 for a list from the mid-sixteenth century, neither of which have anything on the uses of these drugs, nor on medicine, and D. S. Lach, *Asia in the Making of Europe,* Vol. II, book 3 (Chicago: Chicago University Press, 1977), 427–45 for knowledge of Asian botany in Europe.
59. For a dramatic description, see Gaspar Correa, *Lendas de India* (Lisbon: Academia Real das Sciencias, 1858–66, 4 vols), IV, 288–9.
60. See d'Orta, *op. cit.* (note 48), no. 17 for a description of *mordexim* in 1543.
61. *Ibid.,* no. 5, and cf. no. 12.
62. *Ibid.,* no. 9.
63. See especially Boxer, *op. cit.* (note 57), 7–13, Georg Schurhammer, *Francis Xavier: His Life, His Times,* Vol. II, India (Rome: Jesuit Historical Institute, 1977), 203; and M.B. Barbosa and J. Caria Mendes, 'Garcia d'Orta, pioneer of tropical medicine and his descriptions of cholera in his Colóquios (1563)', in *Proceedings of the XXIII International Congress of the History of Medicine* (London: Wellcome Institute, 1974), II, 1258-9.
64. We may also note that d'Orta was followed by Cristovão da Costa, who arrived in Goa in the year of d'Orta's death. Modern libraries often list him as 'Cristobal Acosta, *c.*1515–*c.*1592.' His book in English was called *Treatises on Drugs and Medicines of East India* (1578); the best modern edition is Walter, *op. cit.* (note 26). Earlier scholars claimed that he basically summarized d'Orta, though his book did have numerous illustrations. However, Donald Lach has shown that while he knew of and used d'Orta, the two books differ widely. For example, Costa describes 47 plants, and of these 14 are not mentioned by d'Orta, while nine of d'Orta's are not in Costa. See Lach, *op. cit.* (note 58), Vol. II, book 3, 436–7.

2

Dutch Medicine in Asia, 1600–1900

Peter Boomgaard

Among Westerners involved in present-day tropical health care, colonial tropical medicine has a bad reputation. In their view, it reached only the happy few in the cities, predominantly whites, it was too expensive, it refused to learn from indigenous practice, and, above all, it did not work. On the other hand, until recently conventional historical wisdom had it that the introduction of Western medicine in tropical countries led to lower morbidity and mortality. If we limit ourselves to Java, there is, indeed, evidence for a gradually improving life expectancy at birth between 1800 and 1940.[1] Although other factors clearly contributed to this improvement, there is not much doubt that Western medicine was of some importance. Modern orthodoxy, however, though not denying recent improvements due to Western medicine, emphasizes the arrival of Western diseases prior to Western medicine, implying that European doctors at best made up for the havoc wrought by disease-carrying European sailors and soldiers. This is evidently true for Central and South America in the sixteenth century, Australia and Oceania in the eighteenth and nineteenth centuries, and Africa in the nineteenth and twentieth centuries. The Asian situation is more complicated, and it is unlikely that European maritime contact resulted in similar high death-rates.[2]

These controversies refer largely to the period 1880 to 1940. There are very few tropical areas for which we have sufficient data to judge the effects of Western medicine in earlier periods. Moreover, there are fewer colonies to be studied prior to 1880, and it is often tacitly assumed that Western medicine before Koch, Pasteur and Manson, at best marginally effective in the West, cannot have done any good in tropical areas.

This article concentrates on the period prior to 1880 and deals particularly with the Dutch East Indies (Indonesia). Given the paucity of statistical data, its emphasis will be on – mutual – influences of 'Western' and 'Eastern' medical theory and practice rather than on the effects of the introduction of Western medicine on morbidity and mortality in the East. It discusses the spread of European medical personnel in Asia, and the diffusion of drugs, methods of treatment and theories.

VOC and Netherlands Indies Government Personnel in Asia

During the seventeenth and eighteenth centuries, the VOC (Verenigde Oostindische Compagnie, or Dutch East India Company) sent some medical doctors and a great many surgeons to Asia. Doctors (*medicinae doctores*) were university graduates with a largely theoretical training and a relatively high status. Surgeons had a lower status, lower pay, and a much more practical, artisanal training, focusing on the treatment of fractures and wounds. In The Netherlands, in the course of the eighteenth century, status, income, and training of the two groups of medical professionals started to converge, a process that ended in a merger in the nineteenth century.[3]

In Asia, the VOC surgeons were also paid less than doctors, although the VOC had to permit its surgeons to act as if they were doctors. Only in Batavia (present-day Jakarta), where usually one or two doctors were present, did the surgeons work under the supervision of the doctors. Apparently, employment by the VOC was unattractive for medical doctors. Asia, therefore, mostly became acquainted with Dutch medicine through the activities of VOC surgeons. During the eighteenth century, the VOC had, on average, some 250 to 300 surgeons in Asia, the Cape of Good Hope included, of whom slightly over a 100 could be found in the Indonesian archipelago.[4] This means that some 150 to 200 surgeons were to be found in the VOC 'factories' (establishments) in Persia, India, Sri Lanka, mainland Southeast Asia, China (Taiwan), and Japan. Such a large number might have made a considerable impact, provided that the local medical communities were interested in the skills – such as they were – of the foreigners, and that the latter were willing to share their knowledge.

As a rule, information on the activities of the VOC surgeons in these areas is meagre, at least in the printed sources at my disposal. It is not improbable, however, that a more thorough search in libraries and archives would yield more material. A brief survey of what can be found in the more accessible sources is presented in this section.

We are surprisingly well-informed regarding the activities of VOC physicians in Japan. As the VOC, and after its fall the Netherlands

Indies' Government, was the only European power with access to Japan between 1639 and 1854, the importance of this information can hardly be over-estimated. The story begins in 1649, when a VOC surgeon of the Dutch establishment at Deshima (near Nagasaki), Caspar Schambergen, for the first time accompanied the head of the factory on his annual journey to the court at Edo (Tokyo), residency of the Shogun. He taught European medicine to interested Japanese, probably both in Edo and in Nagasaki/Deshima.

This was the beginning of a tradition that would be kept up, although with many ups and downs, to the very end of the Dutch presence in Deshima. The classes in European medicine produced a group of Japanese physicians who styled themselves the 'Dutch school' (as opposed to the 'Chinese school'), and throughout the two centuries of the Dutch 'monopoly' many of these physicians obtained positions at court. There would always be a surgeon or a doctor present when the chief merchant of the VOC made his annual trip to Edo. During his presence in Edo, the surgeon was often called upon to treat members of the nobility and to discuss medical problems with the court physicians. In 1682, a change took place in the protocol of the audience granted to the chief merchant with the Shogun, and a second, less formal, meeting was convened. Here the Shogun – unrestrained by the rigid rules of the official audience – could indulge his curiosity regarding the foreigners. Sometimes the questions, posed during this second interview, were of a medical nature. Among the annual VOC presents for the Shogun there were often medical instruments from Europe.

Around 1740 interest in European medical science was promoted by the Shogun, who ordered his librarian and his physician to learn Dutch. He also permitted the Japanese interpreters, who always accompanied the Dutch, to possess and read Dutch books, up till then forbidden goods to all Japanese. This more liberal climate seems to have encouraged Japanese physicians of the 'Dutch school' to start translating Dutch textbooks on medicine, of which the first one was printed in 1774. These physicians formed the nucleus of the so-called Rangaku-sha, or 'Hollandologists', who gave the study of Dutch – or rather European – medicine in Japan a new impulse. Many translations of medical texts followed.

The most important VOC physicians to visit Japan were Dr Willem ten Rhijne (in Japan 1674–6), Andreas Cleyer, also chief merchant (1682–3, 1685–6), Dr Engelbert Kaempfer (1690–2), and the well known botanist Dr Carl Peter Thunberg (1775–6). The best-known medical emissary of the Netherlands Indies' Government was Dr Philipp Franz von Siebold (1823–30, 1859–61). Altogether this group consisted of three Germans, one Swede (Thunberg), and one Dutchman (ten Rhijne). Evidently, this was a collection of unusually gifted people, most of them medical doctors, of whom Kaempfer, Thunberg and Von Siebold acquired an international reputation with their publications on Japan. After the arrival of each of these three scholars, interest in European medical science revived among the Japanese. It is clear that one should not over-emphasize the 'Dutchness' of the VOC's physicians in Japan.

After the 'opening' of Japan by the Americans in 1854, the Dutch continued to play an important role in the diffusion of European scientific knowledge in Japan, particularly as teachers in the newly founded schools of medicine and physics and chemistry. This time they were, indeed, Dutch: Jhr. Dr J. L. C. Pompe van Meerdervoort, Dr A. F. Bauduin, Dr K. W. Gratama, C. G. van Mansvelt and Dr A. J. C. Geerts, to name but the most important ones. Around 1880 the Germans took over (again).

Although most Shoguns seem to have been interested in the medical knowledge of the foreigners, they seldom availed themselves of their services. There is a not too reliable story that Willem ten Rhijne treated the gravely ill Shogun in 1675. Almost 200 years later, in 1866, Bauduin and Gratama were, indeed, called upon to examine the Shogun who had fallen ill during a military campaign. There was nothing they could do and the Shogun died shortly afterwards. Finally, I should mention the very personal contribution made by Von Siebold to the diffusion of European medical science in Japan. Oine, his daughter by the Japanese woman Sonogi, became the first female physician in Japan.[5]

Perhaps equally surprising was a not inconsiderable and prolonged 'Dutch' medical presence in Siam (Thailand) in the seventeenth and eighteenth centuries. In 1672 Daniel Brochebourde or Brockebourde, a French-born VOC chief-surgeon, was lent to the court in Ayutthaya to serve as the king's physician, a position he kept until his death in 1697. He was one in a row of experts (cannoneer, maker of gunpowder, enameller, mason, goldsmith) to be sent – at his request – to the King of Siam from Batavia. He had married a local woman while at Ligor, and was therefore fluent in Thai, an asset both to the King and the Company. He was even allowed to treat the women of the palace.

When in 1688 a new dynasty took over, he was not only able to hold on to his position, but he also succeeded in getting his mestizo son Moses appointed as surgeon at the court. Father and son both acquired court titles. When Daniel died, Moses succeeded to his father's rank, title and position, also serving the next two kings and being paid a VOC salary in addition. When he died in 1724, Jeremias, his son by a Mon woman, took over his position as the king's personal physician. Jeremias' brother Philemon also became a surgeon at court. They are mentioned for the last time in the VOC records in 1732, when the two brothers were sent to the VOC 'factory' to fetch the Company's surgeon to cure the king. By then, the Brochebourdes, who had not left Siam since Daniel had arrived there, were probably regarded by the court as Thai physicians, who needed the help of 'real' European surgeons.[6]

Much less is known about the role of VOC surgeons and doctors elsewhere in Asia. I will present the data such as they are, starting with the rest of mainland Southeast Asia, continuing with India, and concluding with Indonesia.

In 1656, a high 'mandarin' of the ruler of Tonkin requested the services of a good surgeon from the Governor-General. Around the same time, the ruler of Quinam (Annam) retained the chief-surgeon Dirk Jorisz van Leyden, who had drifted ashore after having been shipwrecked. The ruler of Arakan (Burma) asked the local VOC Resident in 1663 if he could 'keep' surgeon Nicolaes Bouckens, who had applied for a leave of absence in Batavia.

In India, a certain Master Pieter, VOC surgeon, was lent to the ruler of Bijapur in or before 1639. In the 1660s, the surgeon Gelmer Vosburg stood in high esteem with the Nawab of Bengal, whom he had cured from some painful afflictions. The successor of the Nawab was treated by a VOC chief-surgeon, Jacob Valkenier. In 1663, another surgeon, Jacob Frederick Bertsch, could be found at the court of the Mughal in Delhi, where, in 1680, we encounter chief-surgeon Jacques du Pree, and after his fall from grace – not for a medical but a political mistake – surgeon Jacob van den Bergh.

Indonesian rulers were also interested in the services of the VOC medical practitioners. In 1638, the Sultan of Banten had a Dutch surgeon treat one of his wives. In 1669 the ruler of Sukadana likewise sent for a VOC surgeon from the Governor-General, for the treatment of his Ratu Agung. The Susuhunan of Mataram and his little son, in the coastal town of Tegal in 1677, were both treated by the surgeon of a VOC ship riding at anchor near the coast. Finally, Raja Arung Palaka of Bone (Makasar), suffering from a swelling on or in his nose, was helped by Dutch surgeons.[7]

Given these data, I am inclined to disagree with David Arnold, who stated that prior to 1800, European physicians only rarely offered their services to local rulers.[8]

The pre-modern surgeon has often been ridiculed as a glorified barber, with whom the former originally shared the same guild, but it may well be that the VOC surgeons, often well versed in anatomy and surgery, and not burdened by too many theoretical preconceptions, served these Asian rulers better than the medical doctors could have done. At the same time, it cannot be ruled out that the rulers saw the European surgeon primarily as just another kind of magician, with the likes of whom many an Asian court was well stocked at that time. Given the fact that in the seventeenth century magical and astrological considerations had not yet taken their leave from the medical profession,[9] this was a pardonable mistake.

Turning now to the period after 1800, we observe a rather radical change of scene. The VOC had disappeared, together with the Dutch establishments outside Indonesia, with the exception of Deshima. After a period of uncertainty and turmoil ending in 1816, the former areas under the VOC in the Indonesian archipelago were ruled by the Netherlands Indies' Government, answerable to the king and the minister of colonies in The Netherlands.

It is beyond the scope of this essay to describe the health care measures taken by the government in the nineteenth century. The reader can be referred to the still valuable study by Schoute, although a revised textbook on this topic would be more than welcome.[10] In this section on personnel, it may suffice to say that the number of physicians, which in 1816 had dropped considerably below the 100 mark given for the middle of the eighteenth century, went up to over 300 during the nineteenth century, counting private practitioners and civil and military physicians in government employ. Some 130 of these physicians were European-trained Indonesians. Apart from the physicians, we should also mention several hundred vaccinators and other paramedics, most of them Indonesians trained by Europeans. In sheer numbers of medical and paramedical personnel, Dutch influence in Indonesia had increased considerably.

And how many Asian medical practitioners visited The Netherlands? Apart from one Indonesian in the late nineteenth century, Abdul Rivai, I could only find one Japanese and one Chinese. Nakashima Chosaburo alias Hatono Soha, an early adherent of the 'Dutch school', is said to have studied medicine in the Dutch Republic *c.*1660. In 1709, the Chinese physician Thebitia accompanied Governor-General Joan van Hoorn, who was in ill health, from Batavia to the Republic, where he gave demonstrations of pulse diagnosis and made propaganda for the ginseng root.[11]

Exchange of Drugs, Practices and Ideas: The European Reception

The Dutch did not come unprepared to the East. At the university of Leyden, Clusius and Dodonaeus had spread the knowledge of tropical plants, based on the writings of Portuguese scholars such as Christovão da Costa and Garcia d'Orta, before the first Dutch ships set sail to the Indies. Jan Huygen van Linschoten, who had sailed with the Portuguese to India, popularized the same authors in his famous book *Itinerario.* As a knowledge of herbs was an important element in the training of Dutch doctors, it need not surprise us that they often turned botanist when they reached Asia.

Bontius (Jacob Bondt, 1592–1631) with his *De Medicina Indorum* (1642) is an early example of this tendency. The Swedish VOC surgeon Herman Nicolaus Grim published two books on Asian herbs, namely *Thesaurus medicus insulae Ceyloniae* (1677–79), and *Pharmacopoea indica* (1684). Thunberg, author of the *Flora Japonica* (1784) can be found at the tail-end of the VOC period. Perhaps the two most famous collections, however, were published by laymen. I am, of course, referring to Rumphius (Georg Everhard Rumpf, 1628–1702) with his *Het Amboinsche Kruid-boek* (*Herbarium Amboinense*) (1741–55), and Hendrik Adriaan van R(h)eede tot Drakesteyn (1636–91) and his *Hortus Indicus Malabaricus* (*c.*1700).

Apart from books, collections of mounted dried herbs were also sent to Europe (Andreas Cleyer, Willem ten Rhijne), and VOC ships had standing instructions to bring back live plants. Much of this material ended up in the botanic gardens of Leyden and Amsterdam and their libraries, which reinforced their reputation as European centres of botanical and medical learning. Particularly Leyden, the first university to introduce clinical teaching (in 1636) and a laboratory, and with teachers such as Boerhaave and Sylvius, thus attained front rank among the European medical schools. This situation, in turn, influenced Linnaeus, who came to study botany in Leyden. Many VOC physicians in Asia also corresponded with scholars and learned societies outside The Netherlands, such as the Royal Society in Britain and the Academia Naturae Curiosorum in Nürnberg. The latter edited a journal, *Miscellanea curiosa,* in which Cleyer and Rumphius published their findings and those of their friends elsewhere in Asia (e.g., China).[12] My impression is that European medical professionals assumed, as a rule, that every ailment typical for a certain region, could be cured by drugs from that region: God, who had sent the disease, would also provide the cure. They acknowledged the expertise of indigenous healers in these matters.

VOC physicians were, therefore, instrumental in the diffusion of botanical knowledge from Asia in Europe, thereby influencing the development of botany as a science. It is much less clear to what extent the diffusion of this knowledge influenced medical science and practice in Europe and among the Europeans in Asia. To be sure, new drugs and descriptions of Asian medical practices were often circulated almost immediately after their 'discovery' by Europeans. An interesting example is provided by the spread of drugs against syphilis in Asia and Europe. Syphilis seems to have arrived in Europe with the first Spaniards returning from America, who transmitted it to the French King Charles VII's pan-European soldiery, relaxing between battles in Naples in 1495. It spread, with the returning troops, within a few years all over Europe, and had reached – with the arrival of the Portuguese – India in 1498, Canton in 1504, and Japan in 1512. Before 1500, mercury and arsenic were mentioned as medical treatments, but in 1519, Ulrich von Hutten, a German knight who was afflicted himself, mentioned guaiac (*Guajacum officinale*), a resinous wood, discovered by Europeans on San Domingo in 1508, and for the first time imported from the Caribbean in 1517. In 1532 another remedy was mentioned in Europe, this time from the East, namely *radix China* or China root (*Smilax China*), imported from Goa. Van Linschoten mentioned it as a cure in India and China in his *Itinerario,* and it was used on VOC ships at least since 1610. The population of the sultanate of Banten, western Java, was also reported, in 1644, to use it against syphilis.[13] So we seem to witness the rapid global spread of a disease, owing to the recent European mercantile ventures around 1500, followed by a somewhat slower, but still fairly speedy global diffusion of alleged cures from East and West. In this case, the effect was probably nil, but the rapid diffusion and ready acceptance of foreign drugs testify to a general willingness to learn from faraway cultures.

Another interesting example is the interest in Europe in *moxa* (*Artemisia vulgaris*) burning or moxibustion, used against all sorts of ailments in China and Japan. The first publication on this topic in Holland appeared in 1675, written by a Dutch clergyman, Herman Buschof, who had resided in Taiwan. William Temple, British ambassador to the Dutch Republic, discussed it in 1677. Most VOC surgeons and doctors stationed on Deshima, mentioned above, also reported on *moxa* burning, usually in connection with acupuncture: Cleyer (1679, 1683), Ten Rhijne (1684), Kaempfer (1694), and Von Siebold (1832–52). Europeans seem to have been interested in this practice predominantly as a cure for gout. Already in the 1670s, *moxa* could be bought in Utrecht, where it was sold by Reverend Buschof's son Joan, a barrister. In Germany one could buy 'German moxa', prepared from related mugwort. In the 1680s it went out of fashion in Europe, only to become popular again in the 1760s. Fifty years later it had disappeared. In the seventeenth century the Dutch also introduced it in Indonesia, and in early twentieth-century Batavia, 'heated' *moxa* was still reported as a means to cure haemorrhoids.[14]

Acupuncture was equally fascinating in the eyes of the visiting doctors and surgeons. In their publications, Ten Rhijne (1683, 1684) and Kaempfer (1712) familiarized the European public with this therapy, but it already seems to have been carried out in sixteenth-century Europe. The European public was not impressed, however, and acupuncture was soon forgotten. According to various authors it gained some popularity in early nineteenth-century France. Little did they know that it would be revived in the late twentieth century. Von Siebold tells us about the imperial Japanese acupuncturist, Isisaki Sotetsu, who, after a thorough study of the Chinese classics on acupuncture and 20 years' experience in anatomy as taught by European physicians, developed a better method for acupuncture, which tried to combine these approaches. It would be interesting to find out whether the acupuncture we know nowadays in Europe is this 'new method' or the classical one.[15]

So European physicians – and laymen – reported in writing on their new medical experiences in Asia, thereby encouraging experiments with novel drugs and methods back home. They also experimented on themselves and their European patients in the Dutch 'factories' in Asia. The patients themselves went even further and started to visit 'Oriental' specialists in drugs and health care. Batavia and Banten were busy ports and therefore excellent places for cross-cultural medical comparison. There were of course Javanese healer/herbalists (*dukun*) – often women – who were also good at massage (*pijet*; recommended by Bontius), but also Chinese physicians and apothecaries, Persian drug-sellers, and no doubt Arab and Indian (both Muslim and Hindu) medical specialists.

Thus we encounter in 1681 the German miner Elias Hesse, who, after having fallen ill in Batavia, put himself in the hands of an indigenous healer living outside the city walls. In the same year another German miner, Johann Vogel, got sick while working in the goldmines of Salida (Sumatra). He suffered from intermittent fevers, paroxysms and an enlarged spleen (malaria?). The already mentioned surgeon Grim took Vogel with him to Batavia and treated him there (e.g., with blistering plasters), but to no avail. He then turned to an indigenous healer who treated him with 'powders' and purgatives, which weakened him even further. He was now so badly suffering from dropsy that he did not dare to lay down for fear of suffocating. Vogel then turned to a female Balinese healer, a Christian, who was married to a German. She took him in and treated him with a herbal potion, put him on a vegetarian diet of boiled vegetables (including laxative fruits), following this up with sudatory treatment. After four weeks of this he was cured. Some 130 years later, the British inhabitants of Bengkulu (Sumatra), still sought the services of indigenous healers – in preference to their own medical men – when they were suffering from an indurated spleen. An official decree, dated 1731, testifies to the fact that even the rich European citizens of Batavia availed themselves of indigenous medical help.[16]

As the number of Europeans and Eurasians increased during the nineteenth century, the interest in non-Western medicine grew as well. It is one of the ironies of history that precisely during the period of the great medical revolution in Europe (1860s–1880s), the European and Eurasian lay population of Indonesia was drawn increasingly into the sphere of influence of indigenous medicine. Eurasian ladies, such as 'Njonja' van Blokland, and 'Njonja' van Gent, wrote books – in Malay! – on Javanese drugs and healing practices for a lay public, which were apparently so well received that they went through at least three or more editions.[17] Indigenous medicine, probably slightly adapted, would retain its popularity among this public up to the early decades of the twentieth century. In part, this can be attributed to a lack of European doctors, but to many families who had resided in Indonesia for generations, European medicine was as alien as Europe itself.[18]

The Asian Reception

What did the VOC physicians bring to Asia? Apart from some theoretical notions, which will be dealt with presently, I can distinguish the following elements: hospitals, modern anatomy/physiology and surgery, 'chemical' – as opposed to herbal – drugs (iatrochemistry), bloodletting (phlebotomy), certain notions of hygiene, quinine, and last but certainly not least, vaccination.

Hospitals and out-patient clinics were, at least in Indonesia,[19] unknown before the arrival of the Dutch. Medicine in Indonesia as practised by the Dutch was also much more hospital-oriented than it was back home. This was more a matter of expedience than anything else: the European sailors, soldiers, merchants and bookkeepers who fell ill did not have families upon which they could rely.[20] The VOC and its successor, the Netherlands Indies' Government were, therefore, much more heavily involved in health care than was the Dutch state in The Netherlands. During the nineteenth century, state involvement with medical matters in the Indonesian archipelago would increase with the gradual growth of the vaccination programme and the quinine campaigns against malaria. This form of medical state-intervention was unheard of in Asian countries before the nineteenth century, but was equally alien to the European situation of that period.

Therefore, the heavy emphasis on hospitals and the extent to which the state was involved in health care were neither Western nor Oriental, but a phenomenon *sui generis,* truly colonial in nature. It seems likely that this 'governmental' nature of colonial medicine, particularly in its more coercive aspects, was ill-suited to engender confidence in 'Western' medicine. This was already apparent in the early nineteenth century, when villagers sometimes fled to the mountains and the forests when the vaccinators were on their way. It was feared that vaccination was really an attempt of the colonial government to cast a spell upon those who were vaccinated, in order to make them serve in the army.[21] Nevertheless, it can be argued that precisely these features – emphasis on hospitals/health care centres and the role of the state – are still typical for present-day Indonesia, a veritably colonial heritage.

As we have seen, the European surgeons and doctors were quite willing to learn from indigenous botanists. They were much less impressed with the knowledge of the local healers of the anatomy and physiology of the human body. In Batavia and Deshima/Nagasaki classes in anatomy and surgery for local physicians were among the earliest medical measures taken. It seems that in this respect they may have made a contribution.

The use of 'chemical' drugs was introduced in Batavia by Dr Andreas Cleyer, probably shortly after 1665. Another partisan of these drugs, Dr Egidius Daelmans, author of a popular book on this topic, arrived in Batavia in 1689. In some other parts of Asia chemical drugs were not a novelty. They had remained popular with Arab physicians when Europeans stopped using them after having been discredited by Galen, until the onslaught of syphilis and the teachings of Paracelsus had revived the use of mercury. Although notions of alchemy were certainly older, it seems that the 'iatrochemical period' of Indian medicine (fourteenth to sixteenth centuries) was influenced by the Islamic/Arabic introduction of alchemy and medical chemistry.

Alchemy and the use of metals such as mercury for medical treatment were also known in China before the sixteenth century.[22] We can be brief about bloodletting. It was and remained very popular among VOC surgeons, who applied it enthusiastically to their Asian patients, who seem to have been unfamiliar with the treatment.

I found the first hygiene measures in a report on the Batavia hospitals dated 1744. In particular the expressed need for fresh air seems to have been linked to the miasma theories of the day. This also applies to the measures taken in 1753, when drainage of stagnant water and a better circulation in the canals of Batavia were attempted.[23] The combination of hygiene and drainage would remain on the agenda in the nineteenth century.

Variolation was introduced in Batavia in or slightly before 1779; vaccination came to Java in 1804. An effective vaccination programme came into being in 1815. Smallpox, around 1800 responsible for ten per cent of all deaths on the island of Java, had become a minor disease by the 1870s.[24] The spread of vaccination to the other Indonesian islands was not seriously undertaken before 1850, and in some areas not before 1900. Although the first Japanese work on variolation had been published as early as 1795, introduction of vaccination had to wait until the arrival of Von Siebold, who imported animal lymph from Java in 1823 or 1824. Owing to its poor quality, the introduction was not a success. This also applies to an attempt at reintroduction in 1837. The German doctor Otto Mohnike, sent to Japan by the Netherland Indies' Government, finally succeeded in starting a vaccination programme in 1849. But even then the programme seems to have encountered many setbacks.[25] I am not in a position to judge the effects of vaccination in Japan.

As early as 1764, the Governor-General in Batavia had prescribed the use of quinine, at that time a very expensive drug, introduced from Peru. Not until the 1850s, when the Dutch started cinchona plantations in Java, did quinine become available in large quantities as a cure – rather than a prophylactic – for malaria, which was spreading at an alarming rate. My own impression is that the increased availability of the drug was just able to counter the increased incidence of the disease.

Theory

Moving to a higher level of abstraction, I will discuss the differences in theoretical background of European and Asian medical practitioners. In order to do so, I will follow recent attempts to classify (Eurasian) medical thinking,[26] distinguishing three kinds of systems:

1. Local or personalistic medical systems (primitive or folk medicine, popular and non-scholarly; illnesses often regarded as having been caused by 'personal' agents, such as gods, spirits/ancestors, or witches/magicians).

2. Regional or naturalistic medical systems (scholarly medicine – Galenic/Islamic (Yunani), Indian (Ayurvedic), Chinese – 'great tradition' medicine – based on natural equilibrium models, with underlying humoral-type theories).

3. Cosmopolitan medical system (scientific causality, Western).

I am sure that some scholars will have difficulties with such a crude classification, but in a short contribution such as this there is no room for a detailed discussion of the differences between the Asian systems encountered by the European medical practitioners. Moreover, it is only given here as a framework for the presentation, in broad outline, of the differences and similarities between European theoretical thinking on the one hand and Asian systems on the other.

One could argue that European medical theory, when it was confronted with Asian systems in the early sixteenth century, was not all that different from its Asian counterparts. It was still largely based on the Hippocratic/Galenic complex of elements, qualities and humours (body 'fluids'), which would retain some of its validity until far into the nineteenth century. In this respect, regional/naturalistic Asian medical systems were quite similar. Islamic medicine was essentially Galenic in character and had copied the complex lock, stock and barrel. Indian Ayurvedic medicine was based on three humours (*tridosha*) instead of the four of Galenic theory, and Chinese/Japanese medicine on six (*chii* as governed by *yang* and *yin*).[27] In all these systems, health meant that the humours, qualities and elements were in a state of equilibrium, in which the microcosm of the body reflected the macrocosm of the universe. If the balance was upset, illness ensued.

However, by 1500 the European system had already started to diverge from those of Asia. While the three Asian systems stagnated and even declined during the last centuries of the Medieval period,[28] European medical thinking and practice underwent important changes, starting with the Renaissance and culminating – for the time being – in the seventeenth-century scientific revolution. Important elements in this development were a critical attitude towards classical texts, the increased attention to anatomy and physiology (e.g., systematic dissection of human bodies) (Vesalius, Harvey), significant achievements in surgery (Paré), the establishment of botanical gardens, the growing popularity of iatrochemistry (Paracelsus) and laboratories (Sylvius), growing attention to the natural history of disease or the ontological concept of disease (Sydenham), and a strong emphasis on clinical teaching (Boerhaave).[29]

Therefore, when the Dutch reached Asia around 1600, and when they started to study Asian medical theory and practice in the seventeenth and eighteenth centuries, they encountered an 'official' orthodoxy that had once been very similar to their own, but from which they were slowly but surely distancing themselves. In this respect, Dutch – and probably by extension European – medical thinking may have been rather ambivalent during this period. On the one hand we see Boerhaave starting his classes in early eighteenth-century Leyden with the Hippocratic writings, and we know that bloodletting, a sure sign of humoral thinking, was popular until far into the nineteenth century. On the other hand, European physicians described both the *moxa* burning and acupuncture they encountered in China and Japan as based on the conception that all diseases were caused by vitiated 'humours'. Kaempfer specifically mentioned the similarity to Hippocrates' ideas.[30] Apparently, European physicians were familiar with these notions, but at the same time regarded them as rather quaint, something from the past.

European medical practitioners were also confronted with local/personalistic medical systems in Asia. This is what we usually call folk medicine, with healer-herbalists who are often also versed in 'magical' (shamanistic) practices. As we have seen, Dutch physicians were often impressed by local knowledge of herbs, and they were certainly prepared to copy the more effective herbal therapies, and spread the knowledge of herbal remedies in Europe. In Western criticism, most derision was reserved for the magico-religious side of the indigenous medical practices, such as incantations, amulets, and imitative and sympathetic magic.[31] In other words, the European doctors and surgeons, although themselves in the earlier years certainly not entirely free from 'magical' influences, objected predominantly to the non-secularized aspects of Oriental folk medicine.

An attempt to define underlying theories in pre-modern Indonesian – as opposed to continental Asian – medical practice is far more difficult. Medicine as practised in the Archipelago in the pre-modern period has hardly been the object of serious research. From the glimpses one gets occasionally from the sources, these practices do not seem to differ much from the better documented nineteenth- and twentieth-century healing activities. Although traditional Indonesian medicine has been a fairly popular research topic over the last decades, a comprehensive *historical* study covering the last century and a half, let alone earlier periods, is still sadly lacking, the abundance of sources notwithstanding.

Traditional Indonesian medicine, obviously, contained animistic and shamanistic elements, which it shared with other local/personalistic systems in Asia. Given the historical development of the region one would also expect Ayurvedic (Indian), Chinese and Yunani (Islamic) influences. Greiner, a physician who worked in Indonesia in the 1850s and 1860s, indeed emphasized the 'Arabian' character of medical theory among the better-educated Javanese.[32] My impression, admittedly based on flimsy evidence, is that the influence in Indonesia of the regional/naturalistic medical systems from continental Asia did not reach beyond the courts and the upper strata of the few large urban centres, leaving the countryside and the urban lower classes to the healer/herbalists of the folk tradition. This dichotomy, to a lesser extent also to be found in continental Asia, seems to have been rather pronounced in Indonesia, probably because it lacks a medical 'great tradition' of its own. The almost ubiquitous use of the opposition 'hot/cold', made by Indonesian traditional healers to this day, cannot be read as proof of the penetration of continental Asian 'great tradition' medical theory in the Indonesian countryside. This twin concept – although certainly a well-known handmaiden of 'great tradition' humoral pathology – probably predates regional/naturalistic medicine and seems to have survived in most folk traditions around the world.[33]

It remains to be seen what this state of affairs – the fairly restricted presence of regional/naturalistic medical thinking in Indonesia – did for the mutual perception and influence of Dutch and Indonesian medical theory and practice. It is not inconceivable that the interest in and understanding of Indonesian medicine by Dutch medical practitioners, and the influence of Dutch medical thinking on Indonesian healers were more limited than European-Asian interactions elsewhere in Asia, given the virtual absence of a 'great tradition' medical system that could have mediated between Dutch post-Galenic and Indonesian folk medicine. Without such a mediator, with links to both the folk tradition and the Hippocratic/Galenic theory, the two traditions – that of Holland and the Indonesian folk tradition – may have been more 'alien' to each other than elsewhere in Asia.

Europe and Asia had been connected by maritime and overland trade routes way before the age of Europe's maritime expansion in the sixteenth and seventeenth centuries, and there is sufficient evidence for a 'microbial unification' of the two continents from the fourteenth century onward. There is also evidence that the three 'great tradition' medical systems, already rather similar in several respects, underwent mutual influences during the same period (and before). Therefore, while I am certainly not suggesting that there were no fundamental differences between Western and Asian scholarly medicine, there might be room for the hypothesis that around 1500 they were not as far apart as often is assumed.[34]

As I have argued above, the European medical 'great tradition' was in the process of distancing itself from its Asian counterparts between 1500 and 1700. With the advent of miasmatic thinking, differences may have become even more pronounced. In the nineteenth century, when professionalization of the medical estate in Europe entailed an increasingly strong reaction against lay opinions including folk medicine in Europe itself, European doctors became even more critical of folk medicine in Asia. Increasing attention to hygiene and clean water,[35] even before the great medical discoveries of the late nineteenth century, and the by then completed process of secularization, made for an increasing distance between the European university graduates and the Asian practitioners of scholarly and folk medicine. Nevertheless, in one respect the basic European attitudes towards aetiology of diseases were, in a way, still rather similar to those of the traditional healers: Europeans believed that a great many diseases were caused by invisible miasmata, Indonesians and other Asian folk healers held invisible evil 'spirits' responsible.[36]

The tendency to grow apart was reinforced when, in the late nineteenth century, the 'microbial revolution' (of Koch and Pasteur) turned the medical profession, up to then more a craft than anything else, into a science. Belief in humours and miasmata was on its way out, being replaced by the germ theory of disease, whereas belief in evil spirits was not. Indonesian healers who, by virtue of their greater knowledge of local drugs and herbs, up to then had been viewed by many European doctors as slightly disreputable colleagues, were now increasingly seen as deceitful magicians, or at least as superstitious quacks.[37]

Conclusion

Some 2,500 years ago, written medical traditions in the Mediterranean, India and China came into being and started to distance themselves from local folk medicine. The three 'great traditions' shared some basic assumptions, but they also had their own characteristic features, which they often retained to this day. It would be wrong, though, to suppose that the three scholarly systems and the local traditions from which they had sprung were 'closed' systems. Folk medicine and scholarly medicine influenced each other, as did the three regional systems, albeit in leaps and bursts. Medical exchanges between the 'great tradition' systems followed in the wake of traders, warriors and preachers. In this respect, the meeting between Dutch and Asian medicine after 1600 was just the last wave in a long series.

What set this meeting apart from earlier encounters between medical traditions can be summed up as follows. Dutch – and by extension European – scholarly medicine was changing fairly rapidly, distancing itself from its Hippocratic/Galenic roots, whereas the Asian scholarly systems had come to a (relative) standstill. It was now no longer an exchange between equals, although it was not one-way traffic either. European medicine, developing into cosmopolitan medicine, was on its way to conquer the world. However, local and regional Asian medical systems have been able to survive the onslaught. The price they had to pay for this survival was incorporation of cosmopolitan medical elements. Therefore, traditional medicine *anno* 1995, in itself an ambiguous category encompassing both local and regional systems, is not the same as traditional medicine *anno* 1895 or 1695. As a point of departure for further historical research such a notion, implying more analytical rigour, might be stimulating, particularly in the case of 'traditional' Indonesian medicine, a hazy concept if there ever was one.

Notes

1. Boomgaard & Gooszen 1991, 48–66.
2. Polulin 1976, 124; Crosby 1986, 195–216; MacLeod 1988, 8; Arnold 1988, 4–6. Elsewhere, I have dealt in more detail with the development of post-contact disease patterns and medical care in Asia, particularly Indonesia (Boomgaard 1993).
3. Van Andel 1981; Frijhoff 1983; Van Lieburg 1983; Porter & Porter 1989, 17; Siraisi 1990, 174, 179.
4. Schoute 1929, 106, 156, 283–6; Lequin 1982, 372. An all-time high was registered in 1754, when 379 medical practitioners were employed (Lequin 1982, 73).
5. Kleiweg de Zwaan 1917, 444–569; Von Römer 1921, 78–147; Kraft 1985, 25–54; Beukers *et al.* 1987, 29–40.
6. Ten Brummelhuis 1987, 43; Pombejra 1992, 25–42.
7. *Generale Missiven* II, 64; *Daghregister* 1656/7, 49; 1661, 240, 435; 1663, 6, 165, 425, 664; 1667, 233; 1669, 427; 1677, 274; 1680, 231, 758, 824; Tavernier 1692, II, 537.
8. Arnold 1988, 11.
9. Van Andel 1981, 34–40; Porter & Porter 1989, 193–5; Siraisi 1990, 149–52.

10. Schoute 1935; Elements for such a new textbook can be found in Boomgaard 1986; Boomgaard 1987; and several articles in Luyendijk-Elshout 1989.
11. Kleiweg de Zwaan 1917, 574–5; Von Römer 1921, 85–6; Poeze 1986, 32; Blussé 1989, 87.
12. Greshoff 1902, 12; Von Römer 1921; Schoute 1929, 106–8, 122; Bontius 1931, X–XII; Singer & Underwood 1962, 148–9; Kraft 1985, 42–54; Grove 1992.
13. Kern 1910, I, 158–6; II, 41; Kleiweg de Zwaan 1917, 399–404; Temple 1928, 101; Schoute 1929, 52–3; Saar 1930, 29; Singer & Underwood 1962, 108; Huard & Wong 1967, 98; Crosby 1972, 122–64; Quétel 1986, 9–44, 82; Nikiforuk 1993, 87–109. Schoute assumed that *radix China* was used against beriberi on VOC ships.
14. Ten Rhijne 1684; Kaempfer 1733, 463ff; Von Siebold 1897, II, 82–3; Kleiweg de Zwaan 1917, 210–224; Von Römer 1921, 90–1; Heyne 1927, 1444; Kraft 1985, 45–6.
15. Von Siebold 1897, II, 78–81; Kleiweg de Zwaan 1917, 243; Huard & Wong 1967, 128–30.
16. Vermeulen 1677, 25; Hesse 1690, 66–7; Vogel 1704, 179–95; Heyne 1814, 401; Schoute 1929, 126, 145–6, 205, 244.
17. Van Gent-Detelle 1883 [5th edn]; Van Blokland 1899 [3rd edn]. *Njonja* [*nyonya* in modern Indonesian] = Mrs. It is not always realized that at the end of the nineteenth century the majority of the Europeans and Eurasians in Java often spoke better Malay than Dutch. This would change with the arrival of large numbers of Europeans after the turn of the century.
18. Arnold (1988, 11–12) suggests that, at least in the British colonial world, reliance of Europeans in the colonies on European medicine was increasing in the nineteenth century, whereas my data suggest that in Indonesia this process continued even after 1900.
19. But not in India; cf. Basham 1976, 35.
20. Schoute 1929,1935.
21. Boomgard 1989.
22. Kleiweg de Zwaan 1917, 194–9; Schoute 1929, 159–63, 170; Basham 1976, 21; Mazars 1984, 329–31; Meulenbeld 1984, 48, 56–8; Quétel 1986, 38; Porter & Porter 1989, 158–9; Siraisi 1990, 193.
23. Schoute 1929, 225–7, 246, 259.
24. Boomgard 1989.
25. Von Siebold 1897, I, xvi.
26. Dunn 1976, 135; Leslie 1976, 1–12; Foster & Anderson 1978.
27. Leslie 1976, 4.
28. Bürgel 1976, 53; Porkert 1976, 70; Anawati 1977, 778; Meulenbeld 1984, 48.
29. Sigerist 1961, 331; Singer & Underwood 1962, 110–1, 148–9; Porter & Porter 1989, 158–9, 167; Siraisi 1990, x, 100, 191–2.
30. Ten Rhijne 1684; Kaempfer1733, 463.

31. For medical practices and beliefs in China, see Kleiweg de Zwaan 1917, 27–61; for Indonesia, see e.g. Kleiweg de Zwaan 1914; Kreemer 1915: 69–74.
32. Greiner 1875, 182–3.
33. Leslie 1976, 1.
34. Kleiweg de Zwaan 1917, 134; Huard & Wong 1967, 42–3, 47; Le Roy Ladurie 1973; Basham 1976, 21, 39; Porkert 1976, 72–3; McNeill 1979.
35. Corbin 1982; Luckin 1986.
36. On miasma see Corbin 1982; on evil spirits in Indonesian medical thinking, see Wiselius 1872; Wilken 1887; Kruijt 1906; Kleiweg de Zwaan 1914; Sangkanningrat *et al.* 1927; Van Hien 1933–4.
37. See also Arnold 1988, 7.

References

- G. Anawati, 'Science', in P. M. Holt *et al.* (eds), *The Cambridge History of Islam.* Vol. 2B, *Islamic Society and Civilization* (Cambridge: Cambridge University Press, 1977), 741–79.
- M. A. van Andel, *Chirurgijns, Vrije Meesters, Beunhazen en Kwakzalvers. De chirurgijnsgilden en de praktijk der heelkunde (1400–1800)* ('s-Gravenhage: Nijhoff, 1981 [1st edn 1941]).
- D. Arnold, 'Introduction: Disease, medicine and empire', in D. Arnold (ed.), *Imperial Medicine and Indigenous Societies* (Manchester: Manchester University Press, 1988), 1–26.
- A. L. Basham, 'The Practice of Medicine in Ancient and Medieval India', in C. Leslie (ed.), *Asian Medical Systems: A Comparative Study* (Berkeley: University of California Press, 1976), 18–43.
- H. Beukers, L. Blussé and R. Eggink (eds), *Leraar onder de Japanners. Brieven van Dr K.W. Gratama betreffende zijn verblijf in Japan 1866–1871* (Amsterdam: De Bataafsche Leeuw, 1987).
- 'Njonja' van Blokland, *Doekoen djawa oetawa kitab dari roepa roepa obat njang terpake di tanah Djawa* (Batavia: Van Dorp, 1899 [3rd edn; 1st edn 1885]).
- L. Blussé, *Tribuut aan China. Vier eeuwen Nederlands-Chinese betrekkingen* (Amsterdam: Cramswinckel, 1989).
- Bontius, *Tropische Geneeskunde/On Tropical Medicine* (Amsterdam: Nederlands Tijdschrift voor Geneeskunde, 1931) (transl. of texts, dated 1642 and 1658) (Opuscula Selecta Neerlandicorum de Arte Medica, x).
- P. Boomgaard, 'The Welfare Services in Indonesia, 1900–1942', *Itinerario,* x, 1 (1986), 57–81.
- P. Boomgaard, 'Morbidity and Mortality in Java, 1820–1880: Changing Patterns of Disease and Death', in N. G. Owen (ed.), *Death and Disease in Southeast Asia. Explorations in Social, Medical and Demographic History* (Singapore: Oxford University Press, 1987) (ASAA Southeast Asia Publication Series, xiv), 48–69.

- P. Boomgaard, 'Smallpox and vaccination on Java, 1780–1860; medical data as a source for demographic history', in A. M. Luyendijk-Elshout *et al.* (eds), *Dutch Medicine in the Malay Archipelago 1816–1942* (Amsterdam/Atlanta: Rodopi, 1989), 119–32.
- P. Boomgaard, 'The development of health care in colonial Java. An exploratory introduction', *Bijdragen tot de Taal-, Land- en Volkenkunde,* cxlix, 1 (1993), 77–93.
- P. Boomgaard & A. J. Gooszen, *Population Trends 1795–1942* (Amsterdam: Royal Tropical Institute, 1991) (Changing Economy in Indonesia, Volume xi).
- H. ten Brummelhuis, *Merchant, Courtier, and Diplomat. A History of the Contacts between the Netherlands and Thailand* (Lochem/Gent: De Tijdstroom, 1987).
- J. C. Bürgel, 'Secular and Religious Features of Medieval Arabic Medicine', in C. Leslie (ed.), *Asian Medical Systems: A Comparative Study* (Berkeley: University of California Press, 1976), 44–62.
- A. Corbin, *Le miasme et la jonquille. L'odorat et l'imaginaire social, 18e–19e siècles* (Paris: Aubier-Montaigne, 1982).
- A. W. Crosby, *The Columbian Exchange: Biological and Cultural Consequences of 1492* (Westport, Conn.: Greenwood, 1972).
- A. W. Crosby, *Ecological Imperialism: The Biological Expansion of Europe, 900–1900* (Cambridge: Cambridge University Press, 1986).
- (Daghregister) *Daghregister gehouden int Casteel Batavia vant passerende daer ter plaetse als over geheel Nederlandts-India* (Batavia/'s-Gravenhage: Landsdrukkerij/Nijhoff 1888/1931) (30 vols, covering selected years between 1624 and 1682).
- F. L. Dunn, 'Traditional Asian Medicine and Cosmopolitan Medicine as Adaptive Systems', in C. Leslie (ed.), *Asian Medical Systems: A Comparative Study* (Berkeley: University of California Press, 1976), 133–58.
- S. M. Foster and B. G. Anderson, *Medical Anthropology* (New York: Wiley, 1978).
- W. Frijhoff, 'Non satis dignitatis...Over de maatschappelijke status van geneeskundigen tijdens de Republiek', *Tijdschrift voor Geschiedenis* xcvi, 3 (1983), 379–406.
- (Generale Missiven) *Generale Missiven van Gouverneurs-Generaal en Raden aan Heren XVII der Verenigde Oostindische Compagnie. Deel II: 1639–1655* (W. P. Coolhaas ed.) ('s-Gravenhage: Nijhoff, 1964) (RGP, grote serie 112).
- 'Njonja' E. van Gent-Detelle, *Boekoe obat obat voor (sic!) orang toewa dan anak anak* (Djocdja: Buning, 1883) (5th edn).
- (C. G. C. F.) Greiner, *Over land en zee. Herinneringen aan mijn verblijf in Indië* (Leiden: Noothoven van Goor, 1875).
- M. Greshoff (ed.), *Rumphius Gedenkboek 1702–1902* (Haarlem: Koloniaal Museum, 1902).

- R. Grove, 'The Ezhavas and the Dutch: European constructions and classifications of the natural world of South-West India and the emerging dominance of low-caste knowledge systems 1540–1750' (paper prepared for the Environmental History Conference, New Delhi, 1992).
- E. Hesse, *Ost-Indische Reise-Beschreibung oder Diarium* (Leipzig: Günther, 1690) (2nd edn).
- B. Heyne, *Tracts, Historical and Statistical, on India* (London: Baldwin, 1814).
- K. Heyne, *De nuttige planten van Nederlandsch Indië* (Batavia: Departement van Landbouw, Nijverheid en Handel, 1927 (1st edn 1913), iii parts.
- H. A. van Hien, *De Javaansche geestenwereld* (Batavia: Kolff, [1933/4] [6th edn; 1st edn 1894]), ii vols.
- P. Huard and M. Wong, *Geneeskunde in China* (no place: De Haan/ Meulenhoff, 1967) (Dutch translation of the French original).
- E. Kaempfer, *De beschrijving van Japan* (Amsterdam: Jan Roman de Jonge, 1733) Dutch translation of the English translation of the original German manuscript.
- H. Kern (ed.), *Itinerario; voyage ofte schipvaert van Jan Huygen van Linschoten, naer Oost ofte Portugaels Indien, 1579–1592* ('s-Gravenhage: Nijhoff, 1910), ii vols (Werken Linschoten Vereeniging, ii).
- J. P. Kleiweg de Zwaan, *Denkbeelden der Inlanders van onzen Indischen Archipel omtrent het ontstaan van ziekten* (Baarn: Hollandia-Drukkerij, 1914).
- J. P. Kleiweg de Zwaan, *Völkerkundliches und Geschichtliches über die Heilkunde der Chinesen und Japaner; mit besonderer Berücksichtigung holländischer Einflüssen* (Haarlem: Loosjes, 1917) (Natuurkundige Verhandelingen van de Hollandsche Maatschappij der Wetenschappen te Haarlem, 3rd collection, Vol. VII).
- E. S. Kraft (ed.), *Andreas Cleyer. Tagebuch des Kontors zu Nagasaki auf der Insel Deshima 20. Oktober 1682–5. November 1683* (Bonn: Japanologisches Seminar, 1985) (Bonner Zeitschrift für Japanologie, Vol. vi).
- J. Kreemer Jr., 'Volksheelkunde in den Indischen Archipel', *Bijdragen tot de Taal-, Land- en Volkenkunde van Nederlandsch-Indië* lxx, 1 (1915) 1–113.
- A. C. Kruijt, *Het animisme in den Indischen archipel* ('s-Gravenhage: Nijhoff, 1906) (for KITLV).
- F. Lequin, 'Het personeel van de Verenigde Oost-Indische Compagnie in Azië in de achttiende eeuw, meer in het bijzonder in de vestiging Bengalen' (Ph.D. thesis, University of Leiden, 1982).
- C. Leslie, 'Introduction', in C. Leslie (ed.), *Asian Medical Systems: A Comparative Study* (Berkeley: University of California Press, 1976), 1–12.
- M. J. van Lieburg, 'De tweede geneeskundige stand (1818–1865).

Een bijdrage tot de geschiedenis van het medisch beroep in Nederland', *Tijdschrift voor Geschiedenis* xcvi, 3 (1983), 433–53.

- B. Luckin, *Pollution and Control: A Social History of the Thames in the Nineteenth Century* (Bristol/Boston: Hilger, 1986).
- A. M. Luyendijk-Elshout, *et al.* (eds), *Dutch Medicine in the Malay Archipelago 1816–1942* (Amsterdam/Atlanta: Rodopi, 1989).
- R. MacLeod, 'Introduction', in R. MacLeod and M. Lewis (eds), *Disease, Medicine, and Empire: Perspectives on Western Medicine and the Experience of European Expansion* (London/New York: Routledge, 1988), 1–18.
- G. Mazars, 'Une litterature a explorer: les Rasastra', in G. J. Meulenbeld (ed.), *Proceedings of the International Workshop on Priorities in the Study of Indian Medicine, Groningen 1983* (Groningen: Rijks Universiteit Groningen, 1984), 329–35.
- G. J. Meulenbeld, 'The surveying of Sanskrit medical literature', in G. J. Meulenbeld (ed.), *Proceedings of the International Workshop on Priorities in the Study of Indian Medicine, Groningen 1983* (Groningen: Rijks Universiteit Groningen, 1984), 31–114.
- A. Nikiforuk, *The Fourth Horseman: A Short History of Epidemics, Plagues and other Scourges* (London: Phoenix, 1993).
- H. Poeze (ed.), *In het land van de overheerser. I: Indonesiërs in Nederland 1600–1950* (Dordrecht/Cinnaminson: Foris, 1986) (Verhandelingen KITLV, c).
- I. Polulin, 'Disease, Morbidity, and Mortality in China, India, and the Arab World', in C. Leslie (ed.), *Asian Medical Systems: A Comparative Study* (Berkeley: University of California Press, 1976), 120–32.
- Dhiravat na Pombejra, *Court, Company, and Campong. Essays on the VOC presence in Ayutthaya* (Bangkok: 1992) (Ayutthaya Historical Study Centre Occasional Paper No. i).
- M. Porkert, 'The Intellectual and Social Impulses Behind the Evolution of Traditional Chinese Medicine', in C. Leslie (ed.), *Asian Medical Systems: A Comparative Study* (Berkeley: University of California Press, 1976), 63–76.
- D. Porter and R. Porter, *Patient's Progress: Doctors and Doctoring in Eighteenth-century England* (Cambridge/Oxford: Polity Press/Basil Blackwell, 1989).
- C. Quétel, *Le Mal de Naples. Histoire de la syphilis* (Paris: Seghers, 1986).
- W. ten Rhijne, *De Chineese en Japanse wijse om door het branden van moxa en het steken met een goude naald, alle ziekten en voornamelijk het podagra te genesen.* (bound behind S. Blankaart, *Verhandelinge van het Podagra*) (Amsterdam: Jan ten Hoorn, 1684), 273–91.
- L. S. A. M. von Römer, *Historische Schetsen. Een inleiding tot het Vierde Congres der Far Eastern Association of Tropical Medicine, Batavia 1921* (Batavia: Javasche Boekhandel en Drukkerij, 1921).

- E. le Roy Ladurie, 'Un concept: l'unification microbienne du monde (XIVe–XVIIe siècles)', *Revue Suisse d'Histoire,* xxiii (1973), 627–96.
- J. J. Saar, *Reise nach Java, Banda, Ceylon und Persien, 1644–1660* (Den Haag: Nijhoff, 1930 (1st edn 1662)) (Reisebeschreibungen von deutschen Beamten, vi).
- Raden Ajoe Sangkanningrat, *et. al. Iets over hygiëne in verband met adat, geloof en bijgeloof van het Soendaneesche volk* (Bandoeng: Nix, 1927) (Vereeniging tot Bevordering der Hygiëne in Nederlandsch-Indië, Publicatie No. x).
- D. Schoute, *De Geneeskunde in den dienst der Oost-Indische Compagnie in Nederlandsch-Indië* (Amsterdam: De Bussy, 1929).
- D. Schoute, *De geneeskunde in Nederlandsch-Indië gedurende de negentiende eeuw* (Batavia: Kolff, 1935).
- P. F. von Siebold, *Nippon. Archiv zur Beschreibung von Japan* (Würzburg & Leipzig: Woerl. 2 vols, 1897) (1st edn Leiden, 1832/52).
- H. E. Sigerist, *A History of Medicine. Vol. II: Early Greek, Hindu, and Persian Medicine* (New York/Oxford: Oxford University Press, 1961 [1987 reprint]).
- C. Singer and E. A. Underwood, *A Short History of Medicine* (Oxford: Clarendon Press, 1962).
- N. G. Siraisi, *Medieval & Early Renaissance Medicine: An Introduction to Knowledge and Practice* (Chicago/London: University of Chicago Press, 1990).
- J. B. Tavernier, *Ecuyer, Baron d'Aubonne, Les six voyages de - , qu'il a fait en Turquie, en Perse, et aux Indes* (Paris: 1692), iii vols.
- R. C. Temple (ed.), *The Itinery of Ludovico di Varthema of Bologna from 1502 to 1508* (London: The Argonaut Press, 1970 [1928]) (Reprint Amsterdam: N. Israel).
- G. Vermeulen, *Gedenkwaerdige voyagie naar Oost-Indiën, in 't jaar 1668 aangevangen, en in 't jaar 1674 voltrokken* (Amsterdam: Jan ten Hoorn, 1677).
- J. W. Vogel, *Zehen-Jährige Ost-Indianische Reise-Beschreibung* (Altenburg: Richter, 1704).
- G. A. Wilken, *Het Shamanisme bij de volkeren van den Indischen Archipel* ('s-Gravenhage: Nijhoff, 1887).
- J. A. B. Wiselius, 'Iets over het geestendom en de geesten der Javanen', *Tijdschrift voor Nederlandsch-Indië* new series, i, 2 (1872), 23–33.

3

Race, War and Tropical Medicine in the Eighteenth-Century Caribbean

Kenneth F. Kiple and Kriemhild Coneè Ornelas

In this essay we look at a group of physicians whose approach to disease reflects something of the evolution of tropical medicine in the Americas over the course of several important decades of their history. The group was composed of British physicians in eighteenth- and nineteenth-century West Indies. Some of them were identified with the treatment of British slaves, others with tending British troops; a few undertook both. But all practised under the shadow of war. And although all practised at a time when medicine was moving towards the concept of disease specificity, their writings more often than not reveal a comfortably speculative nature which disdained experimentation. Nonetheless, notions of disease specificity on the one hand, and a wartime demand for immediacy on the other, combined to provide them with some important insights on tropical diseases – and most especially insights in their observations regarding the differential treatment meted out by these tropical killers to whites and blacks.

Disease in the Eighteenth-Century Caribbean

English physicians reaching the West Indies during the eighteenth century could scarcely have been less prepared for what they were about to face. Acclimatized to a temperate island, they were now on tropical islands; accustomed to combating European illnesses, they faced an unknown enemy in African diseases; the familiar faces of white patients were frequently replaced by the darker, exotic countenances of black patients; the complaints of civilians gave way to those of soldiers and sailors; and peacetime practice in England bore little resemblance to the chaotic conditions produced by near-continual warfare in the island colonies.

Moreover, their training, even at best, was woefully inadequate. In part, of course, this was because the state of medical knowledge in general was woefully inadequate – propelling physicians to do, even when they did not know what they were doing. But in part, too, that training provided physicians with preconceptions which frequently blinded them to epidemiological, aetiological, not to mention therapeutic, truths that seem so obvious from the vantage point of the late twentieth century.

And, finally, they were confronted with a rapidly changing pool of pathogens wrought by an ever-accelerating slave trade which was 'Africanizing' the disease environment of the Caribbean under their very noses. The few doctors who left books behind at the beginning of the eighteenth century wrote that the Caribbean disease environment was more or less the same as that of England, perhaps even more salubrious. Thomas Trapham, for example, who practised in Jamaica during the last decades of the seventeenth as well as the beginning of the eighteenth century, could write in his *Discourse of the State of Health in the Island of Jamaica* (1679) that he found that island with even fewer maladies than in England. Similarly, Hans Sloane, a protégé of Thomas Sydenham made the claim, based on his experience in Jamaica during the last years of the seventeenth century, that, save for one or two ailments, he had never encountered an illness there that he had not seen in Europe.[1]

Yet, a few decades later, when William Hillary published the first edition of his *Observations on the Changes of the Air, and the Concomitant Epidemical Diseases of Barbados* (1759), he wrote that the diseases he had observed in Barbados were illnesses peculiar to the West Indies and not ones that were normally found in Europe.[2] One of these diseases, he explained, invariably struck 'strangers', especially those that labour outdoors or 'expose themselves too suddenly to the cool Dews and Damp air of the Night....' The disease was yellow fever, spread by the female Aedes aegypti mosquito which frequently feeds at night. It had devastated Barbados when it first struck in 1647, killing some 6,000 whites; and, again, at the end of the century when it reportedly killed half of the white population. During Hillary's stay on the island the disease apparently smouldered among the new-born whites and the slaves who were resistant to the worst of its ravages, although it did flare up from time to time among newcomers, especially seamen.[3]

An account of another disease to which Hillary gave considerable attention is found in his section on 'The Elephantiasis', which describes filariasis – the infamous 'Barbados leg', also mosquito-borne.

Interestingly, he also noted that Barbados was free of the 'intermitting fevers' which plagued other islands. And he was correct that there was no malaria on Barbados – which has been variously attributed to porous soils, deforestation, and larva-destroying fish that prevented the anopheline mosquito from establishing residence there. We say 'interestingly', because although the anopheles mosquito is the usual vector of filariasis, on Barbados the disease managed to adapt to a new carrier, the culex mosquito. Medical observations from Barbados characterized the disease as one largely of blacks, yet one that was infecting more and more whites.[4]

But, if there was no malaria in Barbados, this was most certainly not the case in most other British West Indies islands – and especially in Jamaica. In the second edition of his *An Essay on Fevers* (1750), John Huxham explained that the most frequent cause of widespread fevers in the islands was 'a moist, foggy, *atmosphere* exhaling from a swampy, morass soil....' Charles Bisset, writing at about the same time, viewed with suspicion a 'nocturnal land-breeze [which as opposed to the daytime trade-wind] comes cool from the woods and high inlands; and is fraught with dense vapours, and other unwholesome effluvia....'[5]

Certainly British physicians were not unfamiliar with the fevers of malaria, an illness that seems to have peaked in its distribution throughout Europe in the sixteenth century. But this was vivax malaria which made one burn and shake and sweat, but seldom killed (although the ghosts of James I and Oliver Cromwell might want to dispute this point). But these men were among the very small minority which vivax malaria customarily claims, whereas the new malaria physicians faced in the Caribbean – falciparum malaria – produced far more virulent symptoms and generated mortality rates many times greater than those of the other malaria types.[6]

It was doubtless the distinctive and dramatic indications of frank cases of yellow fever, falciparum malaria and filariasis, along with the spectacular, if less life-threatening, symptoms of diseases such as yaws, Guinea-worm infection and scabies that prompted Hillary and others to insist that the disease environment of the Caribbean was substantially different from that of Europe. Yet, although these African diseases were delivered to the West Indies in the same vessels that had transported African slaves to the region since 1518, they hardly settled into the region overnight. Rather, they required time to establish themselves, growing human populations to host them, and pathogenic reinforcement from Africa. It was only over the course of the eighteenth century that these requirements were met, as the West Indies, gripped by the 'sugar revolution', imported hundreds of thousands of slaves and generated incredible wealth for their mother countries. In so doing, they became prey, prizes and pawns in imperial struggles that drew huge numbers of European soldiers and sailors into their vortices.[7]

As late as 1700, Jamaica and Barbados had only imported about 220,000 slaves, with tiny Barbados accounting for over 60 per cent of these. Indeed, 50 years earlier, Barbados was the only English island importing slaves, and it was there, where the still mostly white population had achieved a density of some 200 per square mile, that yellow fever made its first known epidemic appearance in the Western Hemisphere. No wonder, then, that Hillary, in Barbados, viewing this disease, was the first to report a significantly different disease environment in the West Indies from that of Europe.[8]

As the eighteenth century progressed, however, Barbados fell progressively behind Jamaica as a sugar producer and, consequently, as a slave importer. Between 1700 and 1810 the two islands imported close to a million slaves with Jamaica absorbing over two-thirds of them. By 1770 over 70 per cent of Jamaican slaves were African-born, and as late as 1817, a decade after the slave trade had formally ended, fully 37 per cent of the black population was still of African, rather than American, birth. And as this flood of involuntary immigrants reached Jamaica over the course of the century, so, too, did a flood of African pathogens – especially as the British did not bother with quarantine procedures as did their Spanish neighbours.[9]

War and Fevers

In view of this, it is not surprising that as the eighteenth century wore on, there was no Trapham or Sloane to any longer insist that Jamaica's disease environment resembled that of Europe. On the other hand and interestingly, James Lind, a naval surgeon stationed in the West Indies during the Seven Years' War, found the disease environment of Barbados, with its diminishing contact with Africa, to be benign. But, he cautioned, this was not the case with the other sugar islands, especially Jamaica, where yellow fever was particularly destructive of white lives.[10]

Yellow fever had slaughtered the bulk of Admiral Vernon's force sent against Cartegena in 1741, and then, in that same year, halved another British force that launched an equally unsuccessful attempt to take Santiago de Cuba. Two decades later yellow fever and, perhaps, malaria considerably soured Britain's success in capturing Havana as the invaders lost 40 per cent of their troops in that summer of 1762.

Lind, who had been a part of the expedition, complained that of 100 men he had landed against Cuba, two-thirds had been lost to disease, and of 17 battalions committed to the fray in its aftermath, the British could not 'muster 600 men fit for duty – they died chiefly of *fevers* and *fluxes*' (his italics).[11]

This lament of Lind found its way into an account penned in 1781 by another physician, Thomas Dancer, entitled *A Brief History of the Late Expedition against Fort San Juan* and was intended as a footnote to Great Britain's then current military difficulties with the French and the Spanish in the West Indies. The disgruntled Dancer had just returned from a secret expedition sent against the Spanish Main – one that was almost totally wiped out by fevers that seem to have been yellow fever and malaria working in tandem.[12]

Shortly after Dancer's book was published, British Army surgeon John Hunter reported that as of 1782 although 'upwards of 7,000 men had been sent there [to Jamaica] during the three preceding years there were not above 2,000 men fit for duty'. He pointed out that the average annual troop mortality rate was about 25 per cent, none of it 'at enemy hands', fretted that there had not been a 'sufficient interval' of time to let London know how weak the Jamaican Command had become, and was concerned that all the dying from disease was dangerous to the war effort.[13] It had become axiomatic in Caribbean warfare that delay in an attack would prove fatal and that if defenders could hold out for six weeks, disease would drive off, or finish off, the besiegers. But, as Hunter made clear, fresh troops from Europe were being annihilated at such a rate that they could not even be effective as defenders. The problem was, of course, that the Spanish defenders were most likely Creole-born and, thus, had already earned their immunities against yellow fever. British troops, by contrast, had had no such opportunity prior to reaching the West Indies with the cost a horrendous one in lives lost.[14]

In 1794 Dr Colin Chisholm published an essay on the 'History of an Uncommon Epidemic Fever observed in the Island of Grenada' which had flared up in the Caribbean the previous year. The disease, which was yellow fever, was scarcely uncommon. But the essay was, for although physicians had long suspected that yellow fever came from Africa, Chisholm managed to trace it aboard ship from the West Coast of Africa all the way to the Caribbean.[15] Unfortunately, the real identity of the disease – soon unleashed on the whole of the West Indies – and knowledge of its African origin were lost as Great Britain went back to war against France and Spain and, in 1793, occupied most of St Domingue. The following year brought more success with the capture of Martinique, Guadeloupe, and St Lucia. For the moment, at least, practically all of the French West Indies empire was in British hands. But the moment was to be brief indeed, for yellow fever had become an unwanted companion of the English troops from the outset, travelling with them from Grenada to Jamaica to St Domingue, and fanning out to infect British soldiers and sailors in the French Leewards and Windwards as well.[16]

By the end of 1795, British troops in the West Indies were dying from disease faster than they could be replaced. In St Domingue, initial losses were between 10,000 and 12,500 men, and by the time the expeditionary forces were withdrawn, some 45,000 to 50,000 men had been lost – mostly to disease. The French had managed to regain control of all their West Indies possessions, save for St Domingue, from the weakened British whose losses among the various West Indies Commands totalled another 30,000 to 35,000, with disease lingering to crush any hopes of reversing these defeats for the British. Indeed, between 1793 and 1796 the British lost 80,000 men in the Caribbean with over half of these to yellow fever. In the latter year Thomas Trotter, author of the three-volume *Medicina Nautica: An Essay on the Diseases of Seamen,* wrote bleakly that yellow fever was so bad that any further campaign in the West Indies 'is now considered as little better than a forlorn hope'.[17]

Shortly after, William Lempriere in his *Practical Observations on the Diseases of the Army in Jamaica, as they Occurred between the Years 1792 and 1797* (1799) expressed misgivings, doubtless held by others of his colleagues, regarding the worth of the Caribbean islands, when he wrote of the 'dreadful mortality' suffered by British troops 'since Great Britain has been in possession of West India Colonies'.[18] But, despite such ominous depictions of the fate awaiting the uninitiated at the hands of Caribbean fevers, in 1802 the French, whether out of arrogance or ignorance, launched their own invasion of St Domingue in an attempt to regain (or retain) the black colony for the empire. Francisco Guerra reports that the pages of the *Histoire médicale de l'armée française à Saint Domingue,* written by the chief medical officer, Nicolas Pierre Gilbert in 1803, indicate no knowledge among the French medical corps of 'the sombre lesson learned by the British'.[19]

It was a costly blunder, for although the French landing force of 25,000 men met with initial success, it then encountered yellow fever, as did each contingent of 3,500 fresh troops that arrived from France regularly each month. Within ten months of landing, the French troops under the command of Napoleon's brother-in-law had seen their ranks pruned by some 40,000, including 1,500 officers – and Napoleon's brother-in-law.[20] By the time of the final surrender of the French the toll has been placed as high as 63,000 Frenchmen, which may be excessive. On the other hand, at that point there were only 8,000 left of the entire expeditionary force, and virtually none of the 25,000 who constituted the original landing force survived. No wonder that scholars have given yellow fever considerable credit for the emergence of independent Haiti.[21]

Black Fever Resistance

Clearly, then, the French failed to learn from the disasters that tropical fevers had rained upon the British. But the British themselves had already begun to learn from their own misfortune, thanks to those physicians to whose reports we have been referring. This is because the physicians in question did not simply take note of the carnage wrought by fevers among Europeans – they also commented on the dramatic resistance black people seemed able to mount against these same fevers.

It was doubtless the differential treatment meted out by yellow fever that elicited most of that comment. Yet because tropical fevers constituted a bundle not easily untangled, it is not always possible to know whether it was malaria or yellow fever that the physicians were observing. Robert Jackson, for example, wrote at length of single tertian fevers and double tertian fevers as if they were variations of yellow fever. Hunter thought that black vomit (sometimes the result of internal haemorrhage in yellow fever) was a symptom of remitting fever (probably malaria). But this was a disease that others called 'ardent bilious fever' (probably yellow fever).[22] In light of modern immunological findings it is easy enough to understand why an observer in Cuba, at about the mid-point of the nineteenth century, when malaria and yellow fever were more readily separated, could write of the black man that 'there is unquestionably something in his constitution or organic frame a something, we know not what, an influence or power of resistance which makes him proof against malaria, and the destructive fevers resulting from what we call malaria when acting on white men'.[23]

The 'power of resistance', we now know, lies in blood anomalies which discourage the proliferation of the various protozoa of the malaria types. Such anomalies were vital to survival in Africa, which appears to have been the cradle of the disease. A blood enzyme deficiency, carried by almost all blacks whose ancestry lies south of the Sahara, provides near absolute protection against vivax malaria;

whereas a variety of anomalies ranging from sickle trait to G6PD deficiency, to a generalized sort of anaemia, affords resistance to the more deadly falciparum malaria. In addition, blacks also doubtless acquired resistance to falciparum malaria in the same manner as others do – by hosting the disease – and surviving it. Unfortunately, however, it requires repeated bouts with a specific strain of the disease just to earn immunity against that strain, which explains why so many whites in the West Indies – with no innate protection – faltered in such an effort.[24]

Unlike malaria, just one encounter with yellow fever provides a lifetime of immunity against repeating the performance and doubtless many, perhaps most slaves, reaching the Americas had already hosted the disease in their (and yellow fever's) homeland. And if not, as permanent residents of the West Indies, blacks also had much exposure to yellow fever, and many of the creole-born must have experienced the mild cases which that disease tends to confer on the young – mild, but still good for perpetual protection. In addition, however, those of African ancestry in the Americas also seem to have been blessed with some sort of innate ability to dodge the worst of yellow fever's ravages, even in those instances when they were clearly bereft of acquired resistance. This was the case early on in Havana in 1649, when creole-born blacks, long removed from Africa, seemed almost impervious to the island's first outbreak of yellow fever – an imperviousness not shared by the whites. It was also the case late in yellow fever's epidemic career in the Americas when in 1878 yellow fever ascended the Mississippi River to fall on a population of whites and blacks previously out of yellow fever's range. Few would have had prior opportunities for acquiring immunities, yet the differential morbidity and mortality data generated by the disease demonstrated in resounding fashion that the blacks had some sort of powerful guardian against yellow fever that the whites did not.[25]

No wonder, then, that European troops, with no innate protection against malaria and yellow fever, and no opportunity for acquiring resistance prior to reaching the Caribbean, died there in a veritable holocaust of fevers. No wonder, too, that blacks, armed with both genetic and acquired resistance, survived that holocaust. And no wonder that the phenomenon did not escape the notice of British physicians. When army physician Robert Jackson noted that 'it has never been observed that a Negroe [sic] immediately from the Coast of Africa, has been attacked with this disease' (yellow fever), the reason was, no doubt, that most arriving directly from Africa had already hosted the disease. But, when Dancer wrote of the mostly creole-born black volunteers of those with 'an admixture of Negro blood' who had survived the fevers that had wiped out most of the before-mentioned expedition to Nicaragua, he seems to have been witnessing, at least in part, the blacks' ability to experience mild cases of yellow fever while whites around them died in droves. In addition, he was probably viewing a demonstration of the efficacy of genetic protection against falciparum malaria.[26]

The observations of military physicians were confirmed by doctors concerned with the health of slaves in the West Indies. George Pinckard, author of *Notes on the West Indies, including Observations relative to the Creoles and Slaves*, first published in 1806, assured his readers that 'Negroes are not subject to this [yellow] fever; when it invades them it appears as a remittent or intermittent type'. One is tempted to speculate that, like Dancer, Pinckard had also observed the blacks' ability to tolerate yellow fever when they did acquire the disease.[27] Shortly after Pinckard wrote, Dr Robert Collins penned his well-known *Practical Rules for the Management of Negro Slaves, in the Sugar Colonies* (1811). In writing of the 'putrid fevers' (yellow fever) he said that 'the reason why Negroes escape their fury, in the worst seasons, and most unhealthy situations, while whites die in great numbers, is a problem which no person has hitherto attempted to solve....' He reminded his readers that the phenomenon was not limited to the West Indies but had also been observed in New York and Philadelphia and proposed his own solution. The problem was fear. In essence, whites had the good sense to be afraid of the disease which blacks did not, and it was this 'insensibility' that saved the latter.[28]

Although Collins hardly carved out a place for himself in medical history with his theory, there is no question that fear of disease and death haunted the world of the Europeans in the West Indies. According to an early nineteenth-century observer, James Stephen, whites were 'seized with terror' whenever they were 'seized with fever' and slaves believed, like Collins, that 'fear kills Bawkra'. Hector McLean, who wrote *An Inquiry into the Nature and Causes of the Great Mortality among the Troops at St Domingo,* reported that disease and the enormous amount of dying that had taken place there had 'filled the minds of every one with terror...' News of the death of loved ones and acquaintances alike permeated diary entries, and the behaviour of planters was certainly conditioned by the threat of death – a threat heeded by those that could afford it – with notorious absenteeism of Jamaican planters the result.[29]

The Formation of Black Regiments

But even as the physicians were indicating fear as the root cause of yellow-fever mortality, and even though they remained uncertain of the respective identities of yellow fever and malaria, and even if their cures were likely to put them in league with the disease in killing the patient, they were also saving lives – thousands in fact. For it was their observations on the different manner in which tropical fevers treated blacks and whites that prompted Great Britain to begin a policy of substituting black troops for white troops in the West Indies – a policy that put black disease resistance to work for the empire.[30]

This is not to say that the concept of employing black troops was a new one. Slaves had been hurriedly enlisted for island defence on numerous occasions over the centuries during the many-sided and lengthy Caribbean conflicts between the Spanish, Dutch, French and English. Indeed, in the case of the Spanish, a large percentage of whites in the population of Cuba made it possible to arm a considerable number of blacks at various times and still leave them a relatively small minority. But the British, themselves a small minority in their West Indies islands, were hardly enthusiastic about arming slaves that hitherto had been prohibited by law from possessing any weapon at all.[31] On the other hand, English troops to protect those islands were in increasingly short supply. Factories lured many young men away from military service as the Industrial Revolution got underway. So, too, did the metropolitan militia. Moreover, England's armed forces had expanded considerably over the past half-century of warfare so that there were more choices within the services. And given a choice, few were likely to opt for service in the West Indies which, given the disease environment, was regarded as tantamount to a sentence of death. Clearly, the use of slaves who could survive in that environment as soldiers would spare the lives of many white troops.[32]

Some experiments along these lines had already been set in motion. Following the fall of Savanna to the British in 1779, black slaves in the area had been recruited into the newly formed 'Black Carolina Corps' which, following the war, had been relocated in Jamaica. Those who chose to remain as soldiers were shipped off to the Windwards and Leewards to become a legitimate part of the British military. In addition, as already mentioned, other blacks (those with an 'admixture of Negro blood') accompanied the mostly white Jamaican volunteers against Nicaragua in 1780. Disease destroyed the effort, but Dancer and others made the point that the mulattoes had fared far better with disease than the whites. And then, in 1782, Barbados, where it had been the custom to use free blacks in the militia, formed the 'Prince of Wales Corps' of free mulattoes to shore up the island's defences.[33]

Fortunately for the whites, such experiments proved successful in that the armed blacks and mulattoes did not use those arms against them – and army physicians stepped up their campaign to make the use of black troops in the islands a matter of policy to ease the 'terrible mortality of white troops'.[34] The campaign bore fruit in 1795, amid chaotic circumstances. On the one hand, Great Britain, the steady enemy of France and alarmed by French successes, felt the need to ready more troops for potential employment in Europe. On the other hand, abolition of slavery in the French West Indian islands, along with French agitation and military assistance, had triggered rebellion in some of the British islands; and all of the British triumphs of 1793 were in jeopardy as white troops were caught up in the hurricane of the prevailing yellow-fever epidemic. The result was a request from London that colonial legislatures form black regiments.[35] For many of the planters such an order at first seemed little short of madness. Great Britain might be worried about the French revolution on the continent, but the British colonials lived in terror of its local manifestation in the slave revolution on St Domingue which they feared would spread throughout the Caribbean.[36]

Yet there was another side to the coin. If the St Domingue slave revolt was menacing, it was also promising in that it was destroying Jamaica's most formidable competitor – a competitor which, prior to the revolution, had been exporting almost as much sugar as all the British islands combined. The British islands could profit immensely from the French misfortune, if only they be protected from the French. Since white troops were scarce and, most likely, would succumb to disease anyway, what choice was there but to employ black troops?[37]

Out of much wrangling and debate and with many misgivings came the formation of 12 West India regiments of black troops with the first formed in 1795, in part with survivors of the old black Carolina Corps. The others, which were to be formed as the need arose, followed fairly quickly. And with the continued presence of yellow fever there was no lack of need. The colonials continued to fume about blacks with arms and, accordingly, clashed with London about matters ranging from their recruitment, to their literacy, to their sex lives. However, they benefited greatly from the role played by the 'blackshot' Regiment in ending the 'Maroon War' in Jamaica and were forced to acknowledge that white soldiers, especially those fresh from Europe, 'sickened and died' in the West Indies while black troops did not.[38]

Such impressionistic evidence, however, was not confirmed statistically until 1838 when the fullness of the wisdom of those physicians, who had observed the Africans' ability to resist tropical fevers, and had recommended the employment of black troops became starkly apparent. It was the year that Army Major Alexander Tulloch published the results of his study of British troop mortality during the years 1817 to 1836. The years in question had been years of peace in the Caribbean, which meant less in the way of troop movement from one place to another where still more troops were congregating – which, in turn, meant much less exposure to yellow fever. Nonetheless, the data revealed that whites within the Jamaican command had suffered an average annual death rate during these years of 121 per thousand mean strength – data, which when adjusted for 'certain omissions', rose as high as 143. By contrast, black troops had died at a rate of only 30 per thousand mean strength. The reason for this remarkable difference was largely the impact of 'fevers' which had killed whites at the rate of 102 per thousand mean strength, but blacks at the rate of only 8 per thousand.[39]

In the Bahamas, which had experienced more in the way of yellow fever during these years, the white death rate was 200 per thousand, the black rate 41 per thousand with 'fever' the cause of 80 per cent of the white deaths. In the Windward and Leeward islands, which had witnessed substantially less yellow fever, the white annual mortality rate was 93.5 per thousand mean strength, while the black rate was again about 40 per thousand indicating how little the presence or absence of yellow fever affected black mortality rates. Clearly the tropical physicians had saved thousands of white lives by spying the blacks' ability to escape fevers.[40]

Notes

1. Trapham and Sloan discussed by and quoted in Richard B. Sheridan, *Doctors and Slaves: A Medical and Demographic History of Slavery in the British West Indies, 1680–1834* (Cambridge: Cambridge University Press, 1985), 19.
2. Hillary quoted in *Ibid.*, 24.
3. William Hillary, *Observations on the Changes of the Air and the Concomitant Epidemical Diseases in the Island of Barbados* (London: 1759; Philadelphia: 1811 edn), 145–6; G. M. Findlay, 'The first recognized epidemic of yellow fever', *Transactions of the Royal Society of Tropical Medicine and Hygiene,* xxxv (1941), 145–6; Robert H.

Schomburgk, *The History of Barbados* (London: 1848), 80, 83, 304–5.

4. Hillary, *op. cit.* (note 3), 125; George P. Paul, *Report on Ankylostomiasis Infection Survey of Barbados: September 4 to November 16, 1916* (New York: 1917); Harry H. Johnston, *The Negro in the New World* (London: 1910), 212; Richard S. Dunn, *Sugar and Slaves: The Rise of the Planter Class in the English West Indies, 1624–1713* (Chapel Hill: 1972), 303; M. J. Ashcroft, 'A history and general survey of the helminth and protozoal infection of the West Indies', *Annals of Tropical Medicine and Parasitology,* lix (1965), 482; Todd L. Savitt, 'Filariasis (elephantiasis among South Carolina Blacks) in the United States', *Journal of the History of Medicine and Allied Sciences,* xxxii (1977), 142; R. Hoeppli, *Parasitic Disease in Africa and the Western Hemisphere: Early Documentation and Transmission by the Slave Trade* (Basle: 1969), 119–22, points out the usual confusion of this disease with leprosy.
5. August Hirsch, *Handbook of Geographical and Historical Pathology,* translated by Charles Creighton, 3 vols, (London: 1883–86) i, 230; John Huxham, *An Essay on Fevers...* 2nd edn (London: 1750), 18; Charles Bisset, *Medical Essays and Observations* (Newcastle–upon-Tyne: 1766), 12.
6. Frederick L. Dunn, 'Malaria', in Kenneth F. Kiple (ed.), *The Cambridge World History of Human Disease* (Cambridge and New York: Cambridge University Press,1993), 859.
7. Kenneth F. Kiple, 'The Caribbean', in *ibid.,* 499–500, and *The Caribbean Slave: A Biological History* (Cambridge and New York: Cambridge University Press,1984), *passim.*
8. Philip D. Curtin, *The Atlantic Slave Trade: A Census* (Madison: University of Wisconsin Press, 1969), 119, table 34; Kenneth F. Kiple and Kriemhild Coneè Ornelas, 'After the encounter: Disease and demographics in the Lesser Antilles', in Robert Paquette and Stanley L. Engerman (eds), *The Lesser Antilles in the Age of European Expansion,* forthcoming (University of Florida Press).
9. Curtin, *op. cit.* (note 8), 140, Table 40; Herbert S. Klein and Stanley L. Engerman, 'Fertility differentials between slaves in the United States and the British West Indies: A note on lactation practices and their possible implications', *William and Mary Quarterly,* xxxv (1978), 372; B. W. Higman, 'The slave family and household in the British West Indies, 1800–1834', *Journal of Interdisciplinary History,* vi (1975), 263–4; Sheridan, *op. cit.* (note 1), 132; Salvador Arana-Soto, *Historia de la medicina Puertorriquena hasta 1898* (San Juan, 1974), 205–6.
10. James Lind, *An Essay on Diseases Incidental to Europeans in Hot Climates. With the Method of Preventing Their Fatal Consequences,* (3rd edn, London: 1779), 41–76, 278, cited in Sheridan, *op. cit.* (note 1), 26. Lind is best known today for his 1754 *Treatise on Scurvy,* but his

Diseases in Hot Climates was a bestseller in his own time, passing through five editions between 1768 and 1808. See Philip D. Curtin, *The Image of Africa: British Ideas and Action, 1780–1850,* 2 vols, (Madison: University of Wisconsin Press, 1964), 72.

11. Thomas Dancer, *A Brief History of the Late Expedition Against Fort San Juan* (Kingston: 1781) 20.
12. *Ibid.*, 43.
13. John Hunter, *Observations on the Diseases of the Army in Jamaica* (London: 1788), 57, 58, 60.
14. John R. McNeill, 'The ecological basis of warfare in the Caribbean, 1700–1804', in Maarten Ultee (ed.), *Adapting to Conditions: War and Society in the Eighteenth Century* (Tuscaloosa, Ala.: 1986), 26–42; for a discussion of yellow-fever immunities see Kenneth F. Kiple and Virginia H. King, *Another Dimension to the Black Diaspora: Diet, Disease and Racism* (Cambridge: Cambridge University Press, 1981), 29–49.
15. Colin Chisholm, 'History of an Uncommon Epidemic Fever Observed in the Island of Grenada', *Medical Commentaries,* 8 (1794), 499–511 and *An Essay on the Malignant Pestilential Fever* (Philadelphia: 1799), 100–1.
16. J. H. Parry and P. M. Sherlock, *A Short History of the West Indies,* (2nd edn, London: 1963), 170–1; Chisholm, *Malignant Pestilential Fever* (note 15), 98.
17. Kiple, *Caribbean Slave* (note 7), 168; Thomas Trotter, *Medicina Nautica: An Essay of the Diseases of Seamen,* 3 vols, 2nd edn, London: 1804, i, 322, (italics in the original).
18. William Lempriere, *Practical Observations on the Diseases of the Army in Jamaica, as they Occurred Between the Years 1792 and 1797; on the Situation, Climate, and Diseases of that Island; and on the Most Probable Means of Lessening Mortality Among the Troops, and Among Europeans in Tropical Climates,* 2 vols, (London: 1799), i, 1.
19. Francisco Guerra, 'The influence of disease on race, logistics and colonization in the Antilles', *Journal of Tropical Medicine,* lxix (1966), 30.
20. Kiple, *Caribbean Slave* (note 7), 168.
21. Robert Percival Parsons, *History of Haitian Medicine* (New York: 1930), 2; Francisco Eujenio Moscoso Puello, *Apuntes para la historia de la medicina de la isla de Santo Domingo* (Santo Domingo: 1977), 31.
22. Robert Jackson, *A Sketch of the History and Cure of Febrile Diseases: More Particularly as they Appear in the West Indies Among the Soldiers of the British Army* (London: 1791), 213, 263, 269; Hunter, *op. cit.* (note 13), 64–5; Bisset, *op. cit.* (note 5), 20.
23. John Davy, *The West Indies, Before and Since Slave Emancipation* (London: 1854), 85–6.
24. Kiple, *Caribbean Slave* (note 7), 14–17; A. V. S. Hill *et al.*, 'Common West African HLA antigens are associated with protection from severe malaria', *Nature* (1991) 352, 595–600.
25. Kiple, *Caribbean Slave* (note 7), 17–20, 161–76; Kiple & King, *op.*

cit. (note 14), 29–49.

26. Jackson, *op. cit.* (note 22), 249–50; Dancer, *op. cit.* (note 11), 12–13, 43. See also Chisholm, *Malignant Pestilential Fever* (note 15), 97, who wrote that 'the disease [yellow fever] did not spread much among them [blacks] nor was it marked with the fatality which attended it when it appeared among the whites'.
27. George Pinckard, *Notes on the West Indies, Including Observations Relative to the Creoles and Slaves of the Western Colonies, and the Indians of South America; Interspersed with Remarks upon the Seasoning or Yellow Fever of Hot Climates,* 2 vols, (2nd edn, London: 1816), ii, 475.
28. Robert Collins, *Practical Rules for the Management and Medical Treatment of Negro Slaves, in the Sugar Colonies* (London: 1811), 259–61.
29. James Stephen, *The Slavery of the British West Indian Colonies Delineated,* 2 vols, (London: 1824–30), ii, 372; Hector McLean, *An Enquiry into the Great Mortality Among the Troops at St. Domingo* (London: 1797), vii; Maria Nugent, *Lady Nugent's Journal of Her Residence in Jamaica from 1801 to 1805* (ed. Philip Wright), (Kingston, Jamaica: 1966), 122–3 and *passim;* Kiple, *Caribbean Slave* (note 7), 181–3.
30. See especially the pleas of Hunter, *op. cit.* (note 13), for the employment of black troops.
31. Roger Norman Buckley, *Slaves in Red Coats: The British West India Regiments, 1795–1815* (New Haven: Yale University Press, 1979), 1–4; Guerra, *op. cit.* (note 19), 34.
32. Buckley, *op. cit.* (note 31), 2–3.
33. Kiple, *Caribbean Slave* (note 7), 167–9.
34. Hunter, *op. cit.* (note 13), 54–65; Buckley, *op. cit.* (note 31), 7–8, points out that Robert Jackson, another who argued vigorously for the use of black troops, had been promoted to the rank of Army physician in 1794, 'the result of the personal intercession of the Duke of York, who, in 1795, became the Commander-in-Chief of the British Army'.
35. *Ibid.,* 16–19.
36. Kiple, *Caribbean Slave* (note 7), 167.
37. *Ibid.*
38. Buckley, *op. cit.* (note 31), *passim;* Guerra, *op. cit.* (note 19), 34–5.
39. Kiple, *Caribbean Slave* (note 7), 169–74.
40. *Ibid,* 169.

4

Resurrecting Hippocrates: Hygienic Sciences and the French Scientific Expeditions to Egypt, Morea and Algeria

Michael A. Osborne

Studies of climate and medical topography provided important foci for the medical and hygienic investigations undertaken by French army physicians during the first half of the nineteenth century. Army medical men and a few assorted pharmacists and surgeons constituted the main sources of medical expertise on the French scientific expeditions to Egypt (1798–1801), the Peloponnesus of Greece, then known as Morea (1829–31), and Algeria (1839–42). A general research programme on medical climatology is extant in the literature produced by all three expeditions, and this programme also formed a mainstay of the French army's medical tradition in the nineteenth century. This genre of medical practice, which I have elsewhere termed 'the medicine of the hot countries',[1] was nurtured by a conjuncture of transformist biological theory and a resurrection of Hippocratic medical theory. The former emanated from ideas about the relationship between the organism and the environment enunciated by Buffon and Lamarck and then revised by several zoologists of the nineteenth century, notably the Egyptian expedition veteran Etienne Geoffroy Saint-Hilaire and his son, the zoologist Isidore Geoffroy Saint-Hilaire.[2]

Histories of nineteenth-century French medicine make frequent reference to medical Hippocratism, especially the careful accounting of the signs of disease found in the case studies of 'The Epidemics'. Additionally, Hippocratic climatic doctrine framed and influenced much of the medical and hygienic work accomplished during these expeditions. This strain of Hippocratic tradition functioned as a medical analogue of cartography. Military leaders held cartography as the most useful and valuable of the various scientific endeavours, and with explicit links to geography and medical topography, the medical doctrine directed attention to the movement and stationing of troops and to the practical problems of army and expeditionary medicine.[3] As an epidemiological method, Hippocratism mandated a careful 'mapping' of disease environments and counselled avoidance of localities, peoples and objects associated with disease.

Throughout this essay I shall employ Hippocratism as a covering term for a cluster of ideas and tools associated with the Hippocratic corpus, a body of writings attributed to the ancient Greek physician. The main foci of the investigation include the Hippocratic nosography of fevers, the idea that health is closely tied to geographical, climatic and 'environmental' constraints, and the notion that the best way to remain healthy is to avoid disease rather than fall sick and suffer therapy. Hippocratism was one of many medical mentalities which informed medical philosophy and practice in nineteenth-century France. Until 1832 every student for the MD degree at the Paris Faculty of Medicine closed his thesis with Hippocratic aphorisms.[4] To be sure, it is problematic to construct a unified guide to the medical art from sayings such as 'Life is short, science long, opportunity fleeting, experiment dangerous, judgement difficult.'[5] I am not claiming there was a pure Hippocratism in the nineteenth century, but I do claim that Hippocratism was a frequent referent of practice. Complete with its notions of humoralism (the idea that disease resides in the fluids of the body) and generalized disease, Hippocratism is sometimes interpreted in the context of internal or clinical medicine as a pole of medical philosophy far distanced from the anatomically-oriented surgeons who by mid-century were increasingly efficient at draining or cutting out the local manifestations of disease. Physicians with Hippocratic leanings shared with their surgical brethren an epistemological conservatism, empiricism, and the impulse to observe and carefully describe the external signs of disease. The healers who accompanied the three expeditions in question exemplified other dimensions of Hippocratism as well.

These Hippocratic physicians distinguished themselves among healers as advocates of a natural historical clinical ideal, a set of techniques that carefully recorded, described and classified the progression of disease within the patient but stopped short of elaborate theorizing and system-building. This general position was summed up in 1819 by the professor of hygiene and medical philosopher Pierre Cabanis, whose writings on medicine contained cautionary aphorisms such as 'Better no theory, than one contradicting certain facts' and 'The theoretical part of a science must be simply its classifications and the relations of the facts composing this science.'[6] Of special significance for expeditionary medicine and French colonial medicine in general prior to the 1880s was the taxonomy of fevers to be found in the Hippocratic corpus, which classified fevers according to their periodicity. Nineteenth-century nosographies, like those of ancient Greece, described classes of remittent and intermittent fevers; genres of afflictions which subjected the ill to (respectively) elevated base-line body temperatures followed by spectacular and periodic rises, or a condition in which periods of normal body temperatures alternated regularly with crises of high temperatures.[7] It was mainly this latter class of fevers, now thought to include the four varieties of malaria, which confronted the French as they disembarked in Algiers in 1830. Although the mortality patterns changed over the century, the medical distinctiveness of North Africa for Europeans lay in the staggering death tolls and morbidity due to the colony's fevers (mostly intermittent fevers but also typhus/typhoid) and diseases of the digestive system.[8]

In colonial and metropolitan medical practice the influence of Hippocratism was especially evident in medical geography, and the emerging specialties of public hygiene and epidemiology. Here Hippocratism was associated with the climatic doctrine exemplified in the treatise 'Airs, Waters, Places'. This Hippocratic tract stressed the careful observation and description of local meteorological, dietetic, and geographic features and their correlation with the health, habits, race and character of a region's inhabitants. Hippocrates had probably used these techniques to apprise itinerant healers of what to expect when they entered a new city or area. French physicians in the colonies constructed their medical topographies and geographies in an effort to solve the riddle of disease. These 'maps', usually influenced by military or paramilitary agendas, were seldom the products of disinterested medicine or science. A good map showed the bureaucracy of colonization, soldiers and settlers how to avoid disease, the key for Europeans operating in the colonies. This sort of medicine later mandated a reserved acceptance of bacteriology among professors and physicians associated with the army medical school at Val-de-Grâce.[9]

In the eyes of the French scientists who observed and recorded the flora of Egypt and Algeria, the botany of these regions appeared at least somewhat similar to that of southern Europe. As Jean-Marc Drouin has noted, the colourful leader of the expeditions to Morea and Algeria, Bory de Saint-Vincent, was quick to liken the botanical productions of Toulon with those of Morea.[10] The French scientists who visited Egypt and Algeria and wrote medical geographies and natural histories were concerned to correct the mistakes of the ancients. Such was the case with Jules-César Lelorgne de Savigny, a naturalist with the Egyptian expedition who devoted himself to invertebrate zoology and also produced a study on the anatomy, habits and mythology of the ibis. Savigny was able to confirm the accounts of two species of ibis in the writings of Herodotus and other classical authors. Thus for Savigny, as for the voyagers to Morea who immersed themselves in the prose of Strabo and Thucydides as well as the Orientalist fantasies of Chateaubriand's *Itinéraire de Paris à Jérusalem, et de Jérusalem à Paris,* both ancient and very recent accounts of natural phenomena coloured 'scientific' perceptions and found a place in the agendas of these modern travellers.[11]

The impressions of similarity to Europe which one gleans from the French botanical literature of Morea and Algeria are not sustained in the medical writings on Algeria. For if the botanists attached to the Egyptian and Algerian scientific expeditions felt themselves to be on scientifically familiar terrain, French physicians in Algeria were both intellectually and figuratively cast adrift, or, to use contemporary terminology, 'uprooted'. Thus their experiences as they encountered what was for them a strange and deadly climate were more akin to those of the physician-zoologists of the Madagascar expedition who spoke of the uniqueness of the island's fauna.[12] Such confrontations had at least two consequences. On the one hand, they spurred physicians to compose medical geographies and scramble for knowledge they hoped would unravel the knot of the great class of afflictions which they lumped together as fevers. With rare exception medicine was without the power to heal, but physicians could observe, diagnose, and issue prognoses in the hope of lessening patient anxiety by telling them what they thought the course of the disease would be. On the other hand, physicians began to scrutinize and question Hippocratic doctrines in ever greater detail. Physicians who saw service in Egypt, Morea and Algeria took the lead in a decades-long bout of hard thinking about the meaning of the term climate and its relationship to human health, race and the settlement of the hot countries by Europeans.

In examining the literatures of the expeditions it becomes increasingly difficult to demarcate the colonial from the metropolitan. The capture of the city of Algiers in 1830 and the subsequent debates over what France should do with this new possession attracted the attention of physicians and scientists who would never visit the colony. Two of these men, the humanist and philologist Emile Littré and the zoologist Isidore Geoffroy Saint-Hilaire, never saw the sands of North Africa. Yet the careers of these two became entwined with debates over climatic doctrine and its relationship to human and animal health from the time they were students together at the Paris medical faculty in the 1820s. Their trajectories underscore the synergistic relationship which developed between metropolitan and colonial careers, biological and medical concepts, and research programmes. Neither man became a practising physician, but their ideas and activities at the core of empire cannot be divorced from investigations of African hygiene and from the European settlement of Algeria.

Although Littré and the advocate of zoological transformism, Isidore Geoffroy Saint-Hilaire, shared republican sentiments and interests in the history of science and medicine, their careers seem to have crossed again only when the lights of Parisian medicine sought to claim them in 1858. Then Littré beat out Geoffroy Saint-Hilaire for membership in the Academy of Medicine but only by a week.[13] In 1830, the publisher Baillière approached Littré and one of his medical mentors, Gabriel Andral, about a new edition of the Hippocratic corpus.[14] The medical historian Erwin Ackerknecht has, with some reserve, associated Andral with a Hippocratic programme of neo-humoral pathology which shared nosological modalities with the teratology (i.e., creation and description of embryological monsters) of Etienne Geoffroy Saint-Hilaire. As previously mentioned, Etienne and his co-author and son Isidore were associated with a current of biomedical thinking that weighed the relationship between the environment and the organism, just as Hippocrates had done. Andral declined Baillière's invitation, but his protégé Littré became the nineteenth-century's greatest popularizer and commentator on Hippocrates. By mid-century his Hippocrates became the proximate source of climatic doctrine, although physicians also continued to refer to the writings of Montesquieu, the English physician Thomas Sydenham and many others.[15]

In addition to being the principal expositor of Hippocrates, Littré's scholarship fed major currents of medical doctrine relevant to the emerging science of hygiene. In the metropolitan context this activity, exemplified in numerous health investigations of prostitution and the conditions of factory labour, probed the relationship between 'milieux' (environments) and their inhabitants. This medicine of aggregates, a kind of natural historical mapping of the conditions of health, resonated with the therapeutic conservatism of Hippocratic clinicians and with the natural historical methodologies of expeditionary science. Hippocrates, as interpreted by Littré, sounded quite like the modern hygienists who specified how diverse elements of the surrounding environment engaged with organisms in the dynamic of life. Littré's intentions, then, were to use history to measure the progress of the present, and marshal the present to reinterpret the past. According to Littré, Hippocratic philosophy consisted

> in the idea he made of the living body, which, according to him, exists by its relations [rapports], and must be studied in its relations with other things. This thought of the Greek physician, completely opposed to that of contemporary philosophers who seek to know the living body in itself, is essentially relevant to hygiene and pathology.[16]

Like Hippocrates, Littré too was sceptical of the therapeutic enterprise. He wrote approvingly of hygiene, the modern science of the 'milieu', as 'both better and more effective than curative medicine'.[17]

Scientific expeditions and the acquisition of a new French empire aided in the renewal and diffusion of Hippocratic medical ideas. Traces of this encounter can be found in Littré's major project of translation. Transmigratory elements permeate Littré's interaction with the Hippocratic texts. That is, the project provided opportunities to engage in armchair imperialism and exotic travel. Indeed, to understand Hippocrates it was necessary to leave, at least mentally, the northern European world. In comments on the text of 'The Epidemics', for example, Littré wrote that French physicians in Algeria

> no longer recognize the pathological phenomena which are familiar to them, and are, above everything else, struck by the extreme dissimilarity between the fevers of the two countries. Thus it is not necessary to be surprised if physicians who practise in our villages and teach in our schools [who] come to study the Epidemics of Hippocrates, are thus found so to speak uprooted.[18]

Littré then found a kind of equivalence between his philological project and the colonial venture. He continued, 'to go suddenly from France to practise medicine in a hot country, or read the observations of Hippocrates, is all one; the impression is the same, the change of scene is as great'.[19]

Army physicians of the era approached the problems of health administration in Algeria with the critical apparatus of Hippocratic climatic doctrine; and simultaneously, Littré affected a rapprochement of ancients and moderns. He attempted to de-historicize, or at least mitigate, the antiquity of his subject by rendering a Hippocrates he hoped would 'be read and understood as a contemporary book'.[20] More specifically, Littré de-historicized Hippocrates through frequent comments on current medical practice, retrospective diagnosis, and by assigning modern names to the afflictions mentioned by Hippocrates and his associates. In prose which must have found considerable favour with the empirics, Littré explained that although the progress of the medical art had improved upon Hippocrates, his method 'and the method [of modern medicine] do not differ in their essence because they are, the one and the other, the experimental method'.[21]

The editing and translation of Hippocrates consumed Littré for more than two decades. The very length of the work also meant that each volume, from the first (1839) instalment, which won him entry into the Académie des Inscriptions et Belles Lettres, to the tenth and last (1861), was subject to intensive scrutiny, comment and review. In numerous prefaces, introductions, advertisements, and retrospective remarks stretching across the 6,442-page monument of French and Greek, Littré credited, chided and answered a host of critics and admirers as he interjected his own summaries of the Hippocratic arguments. Events and physicians in Algeria and other hot countries of European interest participated in this dialogue, and they, in turn, were important to Littré's understanding of Hippocrates.

Imbued with the spirit of positivism in the 1840s, Littré admired Hippocrates for liberating medicine from the regime of the priests.[22] Littré did not call for a return to ancient medicine. The world itself was much changed, and contemporary medicine faced what the ancients had not: 'the entire globe open to explorations, sundry races and their mixtures, extensive navigations, distant colonizations, demographic studies; all this forms a vast totality which modern science reworks....'[23] Thus the Hippocrates resurrected by Littré functioned as the progressive symbol of common sense and resonated with the utilitarian sensibilities of the scientists who worked on the periphery of empire. The ancient physician of Cos had explicitly compared the environments for medical practice in Europe and Asia, paying special attention to physical and moral differences of the inhabitants, and correlating them with the physical nuances of climates and soils. For expeditionary physicians, Hippocrates appeared as a sort of bridge – one of the few – between the metropolitan world of their medical training and the new world of sand and fevers encountered in Egypt and Algeria.

Contemporary colonial knowledge provided Littré with information essential to his project. Especially relevant seemed the reports of French army physicians in the nascent colony of Algeria and the disastrous experiences recorded by the Morea expedition. Dr François Clément Maillot, for example, who collected several observations from hospitals in Algiers and Bône and would later become the colony's leading advocate of quinine in fever therapy, wrote of intermittent fevers. Littré used these observations to explicate clinical observations in the Hippocratic corpus.[24]

Maillot's experience in the colony exemplifies the feeling of being uprooted and cast adrift. For example, in confronting what both he and Hippocrates classed as false continuous fevers (probably typhoid) Maillot wrote that 'We search in vain to find, in that which is special about this illness, a few analogies ... [to the class of typhoid fevers]'. The symptomatology of typhoid, the greatest single cause of death for French soldiers in Algeria in the nineteenth century, was familiar to military physicians who practised in the metropolis. Yet the conditions of medical practice overseas required a reworking of metropolitan medical knowledge and art. Maillot, for example, concluded that in Algeria typhoid sufferers entered a state of 'chills' or cold shivering, a condition 'nearly unknown outside of warm and swampy countries'.[25]

Maillot's sense of being cast adrift was not unique. Many military physicians of the first half of the nineteenth century shared his sentiments. Metropolitan medicine was not working, and as if practitioners did not have enough to do, the Army began to describe and make explicit its medical and sanitary failures by compiling statistical indicators of health and non-health. The numbers showed what the medical community already knew: French soldiers had never prospered on the eastern and southern shores of the Mediterranean. In Algeria, the men were dying in droves, and the major cause was disease, primarily fevers, and not enemy fire. In some years during the 1830s, for example, the chances of a young soldier meeting his death while serving in Algeria were eight times greater than members of his metropolitan cohort.[26]

Having described the conceptual apparatus of Hippocratism, and signalled some effects of the medical work of the expeditions on Littré's Hippocrates, it remains to examine in turn the medical lessons of the three scientific expeditions which form our subject of inquiry. Let us commence with Egypt.

Mapping the Ecology of Disease in Egypt

The two key physicians of Bonaparte's Egyptian expedition had followed their leader to the Levant from Italy. The Surgeon-General, Dominique Larrey, and the chief Physician-General, René Desgenettes, produced several studies on the health of the Egyptian army. They describe the disease ecology of Egypt as displaying a mixture of European and local afflictions. Thus, in comparison to Maillot and the physicians of the 1830s, their narratives seem less 'uprooted' and more linked to European medical experiences with the Napoleonic armies. While confronted with the usual 'dysenteries' among the troops, the physicians wrote with great concern about outbreaks of smallpox and that old scourge of the East, plague. Yet even with plague, both men speculated that Egypt might even be a healthier place for military operations than Europe. Larrey, for example, drew attention to the climate of the Nile Valley and noted how wounds healed quickly in the hot and dry environment while gout, scabies and other diseases common to the French troops seemed to disappear. Desgenettes even calculated that the Egyptian army was actually much healthier than its cohort in Europe.[27]

Egypt seemed nonetheless replete with diseases exotic and common. Larrey, whose surgical training led to a localistic conceptualization of disease and speculations about 'germs' and 'viruses', described many diseases seldom encountered in Europe including yellow fever, leprosy and elephantiasis.[28] The lessons of the health history of the Egyptian campaign would be recounted by Larrey to his students at the Army's postgraduate medical school at Val-de-Grâce in the 1820s. About 4,500 men had perished or fallen gravely ill during the campaign, and disease rather than enemy fire put all but 400 of this total on the sick-list. In one disaster alone, the plague had flared up and claimed 64 health officers. Clearly, scientists and soldiers of future expeditions needed to take special precautions against the health dangers posed by activity in the hot countries of the Mediterranean Basin. Curiously, the gravity of these dangers was reflected neither in the organization of the Institute of Egypt, which had no medical section, nor in the few publications on hygiene and medicine in the volumes of the *Description d'Egypte* which totalled only a small fraction of the 126 separate memoirs.[29] As Numa Broc has shown, French explorers of the nineteenth century were remarkable for the diversity of their scientific specialties, but physicians accounted for only ten of the 151 members of the scientific and artistic commission which visited Egypt.[30]

Desgenettes, with interests in hygiene, demography and epidemiology, gained his MD at the font of eighteenth-century medical Hippocratism, the medical school at Montpellier. He would later broadcast his medical theories from the chair of hygiene at the Paris Faculty of Medicine from 1830 to 1837. Desgenettes stands as an exemplar of a practitioner who lived a significant part of his career practising and writing memoirs about the 'medicine of the hot countries'. In Egypt, Desgenettes conceived of a medical and topographic study of the old city of Cairo and constructed necrological tables. Such a strategy provided the army with a guide for the simultaneous avoidance of both disease and areas where troops might be attacked.

The experiences of the Egyptian expedition caused French military physicians to further investigate the diseases of the southern and eastern Mediterranean Basin which were known to be among the hot or warm countries of the world. Their efforts spoke to the necessities of military and expedition life and articulated with a broad range of ongoing sanitary and civil engineering concerns. As a general tendency the Hippocratic physicians placed considerable emphasis on quarantine and the avoidance of disease rather than on therapy. They also opened the possibility for European colonization of new territories by insisting on the flexibility of European physiology – the so-called cosmopolitanism of the European race – and on the ability to acquire qualities of resistance to morbid climates similar to those perceived in indigenous populations.

Subsequent scientific ventures to Morea and Algeria were modelled after the Egyptian expedition. In Morea and Algeria, as well as on expeditions to Greenland (1835–6) and Abyssinia (1839–43), medicine and medical men were considered necessary for the scientists to accomplish their tasks, but medical activities had a rather low scientific status compared to the work of natural history, physical geography and archaeology. Leading the way in Morea and Algeria was Jean Baptiste Georges Marie Bory de Saint-Vincent. An avowed materialist and a supporter and improver of Lamarck's theories of biological transformation, Bory de Saint-Vincent spent time in exile and lived in a cave in Holland before becoming a general in the French army and head of the historical division at the Ministry of War.[31] His organization of the Algerian expedition into sections based on geography rather than disciplines ran against narrowly specialized and thematic treatments.[32]

In comparison to the expeditions to Egypt and Algeria, the Morea venture was small in scale and quite different in scope and intention. As was the case with Egypt, medicine was not well represented in the formal activity of the Morea expedition. The commission which visited the peninsula was divided into sections for the physical sciences, archaeology, and architecture and sculpture, a structure which mimicked the composition of the metropolitan bodies involved in its organization – the Académies des Sciences, Inscriptions, and Beaux-Arts. Yet there is no denying that disease, health and medical geography were factors in the conduct and especially the fate of the expedition. Bory de Saint-Vincent, who recounted how he survived the Morea experience with dark glasses to guard against the sun and substantial doses of quinine, claimed that the incidence of fevers reduced the time for mapping, collection and examination of objects to about six months. Health considerations also forced members of the commission to avoid pitching its tents near swampy areas.[33] Bory de Saint-Vincent described Greece as a degraded place with degraded and wretched people in need of restoration and the benefits of French civilization. Evidence of just how far Greece had fallen was to be seen in the tortures visited upon the expedition members which included repeated attacks of fleas, other pests, and a high incidence of scabies. His impressions of Greece echoed Chateaubriand's depictions of the Orient, the two regions providing exemplars of what happened when great civilizations suffered reduction to the savage state.[34] In terms of its general disease ecology and geographical formations, Greece was likened to Italy, southern France and Spain.[35] In Morea, as in Egypt, epidemic diseases visited members of the expedition. Bory de Saint-Vincent called the fevers which struck down the expedition near Helos a visitation by 'new Harpies'. Ever the romantic popularizer of his own triumphs, he told the sad tale of struggle and death in great detail.[36] By the time of the organization of the Algerian expedition in the late 1830s, the eastern Mediterranean was distinguished in military medical circles as a region of fevers and plague.

Reworking Algeria: French Hygiene and the Civilizing Process

J. A. N. Périer, the army physician charged with writing the medical sciences report for the scientific expedition to Algeria in the late 1830s, seems also to have been cast adrift and uprooted. Unsure of, but unwilling to let go of, current metropolitan medical techniques, Perier exemplified several traits of the Hippocratic medical mentality and agreed with the medical philosopher Cabanis who had noted that just as natural history required a good physical geography, so too 'the science of man needed a good medical geography'.[37] Although his ideal science of hygiene rested on understanding the physical constitution of a locality and the modifications that area's uniqueness exerted on human well being, he offered only a first instalment to a complete medical geography of the colony. This task was central to the work of the military and to settlement of the Maghreb by Europeans.

With its conceptual debt to Greek climatic doctrine, its methodological heritage drawn from natural history, and perhaps, too, because the object of the writer's gaze, North Africa, had once played a much grander role in the political and economic life of the Mediterranean Basin, Périer's medical geography was no less a project of resurrection, reworking and restoration than Littré's Hippocrates. Périer portrayed previous empires – the French, Persian, Egyptian and Syrian – as having fallen into degraded states. The fruit of this process, depicted by Périer in terms which evoked Greek ideals of balance and proportionality in rather macabre terms, was of course a weakening of 'human industry' to combat disease. Disease, both endemic and epidemic, prospered or faltered 'according to the retrograde or progressive development of civilization'.[38]

Périer's notions of barbarism and civilization require further comment. Périer, who as a physician did not treat native political organization in detail, mentions barbarism just once as part of the collage of incessant variety which made up the nascent colony. Barbarian behaviour connoted the actions of nomadic peoples, bands of humanity without agriculture rather than those lacking a specific political regime. The peoples of the Tell, for example, are described as having some elements of civilization. These tribes with different physical, intellectual and moral characteristics, lived under aristocratic, democratic or theocratic regimes. But organized or not, Périer paints the colony as fallen, diseased and besotted with ignorance. In short, the Algerians were in need of the French and the institutions of their civilization, especially scientific agriculture and medicine. It rests with France, wrote Périer, to 'pick up Algeria from its fall and to restore it to its ancient glory; ... hygiene signals the sources of disease: may the higher administration neglect nothing to hasten the decontamination. This honour is reserved, above all, to the ploughshare; to cultivate, is this not to sanitize?'[39]

The first chapter of Périer's two-volume survey, composed at the same time Littré was penning his great monument of medical history, is peppered with citations to Hippocrates, both to Littré's edition and one by Charles Victor Daremberg. Périer also cited Herodotus, Pliny, Strabo and assorted other ancients, mostly Greek but also Roman. In form and content the volumes on hygiene rework and update Hippocrates' 'Airs, Waters, Places'; a major difference being that Périer adds the rubric of wood, an important economic, sanitary and technological preoccupation of the French throughout the colonial period. Trees were important for settlement. Native cork oaks provided the French with bottle corks for wine and wall covering for the bedrooms of hypochondriac writers in Paris such as Marcel Proust. Clumps of introduced eucalyptus, those symbols of France's power to refashion Barbary, provided firewood, telegraph poles, railway ties, and had the added advantage of drying up swamps and reducing the incidence of fevers. Viewed from Périer's Hippocratic perspective, planting trees was essential to remediation of the environment and to the improvement of human health. Because trees improved the constitution of the atmosphere and locality, they also exerted beneficial effects on the cleanliness of the air, the regularity of the seasons and the fertility of the soil.[40]

Spinning out from the conceptual core of Hippocratic medical geography were such interwoven questions as could Europeans adapt to the conditions of life in the colonies? Failing the real, sustained and heritable physiological adaptation of Europeans to these exotic disease regimes, could they at least avoid the major health threats by adopting new rules of diet, dress or behaviour, or by Europeanizing the African environment through sanitary projects and the introduction of modern systems of cultivation? For Périer and others, the answers lay with a prudent mixture of climatic and racial hygiene.

According to Périer, the dynamic of human health oscillated within certain limits. Individuals and the various races of humanity possessed an innate texture or bodily constitution which favoured health in certain locales and predisposed one to illness in others. The key to adaptation for Europeans in the new climatic circumstances of North Africa was to become like the natives in some respects; to become assimilated to a lifestyle like the indigenous peoples. The European races could only 'take root', he wrote, through the 'instrumentality of the profound modifications which result from crossing with the natives'.[41] Périer thought that those who issued from the union of European and African would most certainly tolerate the hot temperatures of Algeria more easily than their European forebears. Still, a complete adaptation to local disease regimes, in other words the specific miasms, infections and poisons of each village and town, would remain problematic. Sometimes native peoples, especially native troops fighting in the French army, appeared to sustain the seasonal fevers of Algeria better than Europeans. At other times natives suffered greater losses than the Europeans.

In addition to intermarriage, the European who became acclimatized to Algeria became like the natives in very material ways. After several years he donned the 'colour of the native, accepted their customs and even, to a certain degree, the direction of [their] ideas'. In short the European 'lost something of himself which he replaced by something to which he is assimilated....' Périer viewed this new physiological state, a sort of harmonization of the organism with the exterior world, as a necessity for sustained European presence in the colony. Becoming like the natives was to a degree necessary, in matters of health and lifestyle, although he feared that if the process went too far the French would become like the lotus eaters of

Homer's *Odyssey* and forget their origins.[42]

Périer speculated, as did his fellow army physician, Dr J. C. M. Boudin, a veteran of the fevers of Morea, that residence in Algeria and contracting a mild case of the fevers might have the health benefit of preserving one against tuberculosis and the other diseases common to Europe. Thus the physiological changes wrought by acclimatization to the climate of North Africa might confer immunity to some diseases. This idea replayed Greek notions of balance, and Périer was quick to cite cases described by Hippocrates where afflictions such as haemorrhoids, which removed moisture from the body, preserved the patient from other 'wet' diseases such as pleurisy, pneumonia and certain classes of ulcers.[43]

Unlike the literature of the Morea expedition, and to a lesser extent that of Egypt, Périer's study of Algeria was replete with recommendations for settlement policy. His hygienic doctrine was one of extreme geographic localization. That is, the fevers of the colony came in 'infinite varieties', according to the location of their appearance, and therefore Europeans who became acclimatized did so only to the climate and disease regimes of a certain region or city, be it Oran, Bône or Algiers. Thus troops and, by implication, settlers needed to reside as long as possible in one place and not move around.[44] Périer's assimilationist programme of the 1830s and 1840s testifies to the persistence of the Hippocratic medical ideals which informed the medical work of all three scientific expeditions. The future of European settlement in North Africa rested on a fusion of blood and ideas, and the cornerstone of this effort would be a racial mixing destined to provide future generations of Europeans with something those of the 1830s had lacked, a physiological 'constitution in perfect relationship with the climate'.[45] Until this mixed race of Europeans and natives grew to maturity, Europeans would need to concentrate on avoiding disease through sober and moderate behaviours, and on the removal of the climatic threat through the 'progressive sanitation of the soil which will revolutionize in greater and greater degree the nature of the climate'.[46] The mixture of ideas, which for Périer meant instructing the indigenous peoples in French and the tenets of French civilization, contained few vestiges of reciprocity and no positive valuation of things foreign. Thus health was something the Europeans wished to appropriate, while in general indigenous knowledge was held in low esteem. Western medicine itself provides a case in point. When indigenous medical knowledge deserved study, it was less to add to the canon of Western medicine than to try to reach the local empiric physicians and convince them of the superiority of French medical technique.[47]

By the 1860s Périer had reversed his stance on the necessity of intermarriage and shifted to the position that racial mixing was not necessary for the progress of the human races.[48] His politics, now diffused through the forum of the Société d'anthropologie de Paris, argued that association (i.e., segregation of European and indigenous peoples), rather than assimilation, ought to guide French relations with the subject peoples of the colonies and blacks in general. This move toward associationism on racial and medical grounds predates by some three decades the associationist consensus in French colonial policy of the 1890s.[49] It coincided with a growing realization that hygienic measures, civil engineering and the extension of European agriculture had fashioned Algeria into a relatively healthy place for Europeans. Indeed, by 1866 a study commission of the British War Office praised the sanitary improvements of the French in Algeria, particularly 'deep ploughing, cropping, and drainage' as the surest means to battle malaria in any warm climate colony, including India.[50]

The medical work of the expeditions left an imprint on the scientific and medical worlds of the French metropolis. On the whole, the medicine of the expeditions remained subservient to military needs as later, in Algeria, to settlement policy. Still, Paris and commanding officers did not always give clear directives. Thus the relationship between colonial knowledge and metropolitan activities was dynamic and continually re-negotiated. Within the expeditionary context, Hippocratic medicine, suitably resurrected and de-historicized, served as an instrument of French colonialism and imperialism.[51] French physicians continued to use the medical database created by the expeditions whenever they debated the nature of climates and the extent of the physiological adaptation of Europeans in the hot countries. And this debate, of course, continued into the early years of this century.

Notes

I wish to thank Marie-Noëlle Bourguet, Sharon Farmer, Anita Guerrini, Lisa Kallet-Marx, Anne Marie Moulin, Ann Moyer, Daniel Nordman and Paolo Palladino for comments on various versions of this paper. Research for this project was supported by grants from the Faculty Senate and the Interdisciplinary Humanities Center of the University of California, Santa Barbara.

1. M. A. Osborne, 'French military epidemiology and the limits of the laboratory: The case of Louis-Félix-Achille Kelsch', in A. Cunningham and P. Williams (eds), *The Laboratory Revolution in*

Medicine (Cambridge: Cambridge University Press, 1992), 189–208.

2. See 'The scientific basis of acclimatization in France', Ch. 3 of my *Nature, the Exotic, and the Science of French Colonialism* (Bloomington: Indiana University Press, 1994).
3. Bernard Lepetit, 'Missions scientifiques de expéditions militaires: Remarques sur des modalités d'articulation', paper delivered at the seminar 'L'invention scientifique de la Mediterranée', UFR de Géographie, Histoire, Sciences de la Société, University of Paris VII, November 1992.
4. E. H. Ackerknecht, *Medicine at the Paris Hospital, 1794–1848* (Baltimore: Johns Hopkins Press, 1967), 5.
5. Quoted from the *Aphorisms* in M. C. Howatson (ed.), *Oxford Companion to Classical Literature,* 2nd edn, (Oxford: Oxford University Press, 1989), 279.
6. Ackerknecht, *op. cit.* (note 4), 6, quoting from, respectively, *Du dégré de certitude de la médecine,* 3rd edn, (Paris: 1819), 7; *Coup d'oeil sur les révolutions et sur la réforme de la médecine* (Paris: 1804), 271.
7. D. G. Carlson, *African Fever: A Study of British Science, Technology and Politics in West Africa, 1787–1864* (Canton, Ma.: Science History Publications, 1984), 27.
8. P. D. Curtin, *Death by Migration: Europe's Encounter with the Tropical World in the Nineteenth Century* (Cambridge: Cambridge University Press, 1989), 188–93.
9. Osborne, *op. cit.* (note 1).
10. J.-M. Drouin, 'Bory de Saint-Vincent et la géographie botanique', paper delivered at the seminar 'L'invention scientifique de la Mediterranée', UFR de Géographie, Histoire, Sciences de la Société, University of Paris VII, February 1993.
11. C. C. Gillispie, 'Scientific aspects of the French Egyptian expedition, 1798–1801', *Proceedings of the American Philosophical Society,* cxxxiii (1989), 458–9; *Expedition scientifique de Morée. Section des sciences physiques, I, Relation du voyage,* by Bory de Saint-Vincent (Paris: F. G. Levrault, 1836), 22.
12. J. Lemure, *Madagascar: L'expédition au point de vue médicale et hygienique* (Paris: J. B. Baillière, 1896).
13. S. Aquarone, *The Life and Works of Emile Littré* (Leyden: Sythoff, 1958), 85.
14. J. Jouanna, 'Littré, éditeur et traducteur d'Hippocrate', *Revue de synthèse,* cvi–cviii (1982), 286; *idem, Hippocrate* (Paris: A. Fayard, 1992), 85.
15. Ackerknecht, *op. cit.* (note 4), 106–7, 167–8. Jouanna cites several other editions of Hippocrates completed in nineteenth-century Europe. Important for the French context was the work of Charles Victor Daremberg on Greek and Roman medicine. See his *Galien* (Paris: J. B. Baillière, 1854–6) and *Etat de la médicine entre Homère et Hippocrate* (Paris: Didier, 1869).

16. Littré, *Oeuvres complètes d'Hippocrate,* (Paris: J. B. Baillière, 1839–61), Vol. I, 464.
17. Littré, *La Science au point de vue philosophique* (Paris: Didier, 1873), 271.
18. Littré, *op. cit.* (note 16), Vol. II, 564.
19. *Ibid.,* 564–5.
20. Cited by Jouanna, *op. cit.* (note 14), 296, from *Oeuvres complètes,* Vol. I, ix.
21. Littré, 'Exposé sommaire de la doctrine médicale d'Hippocrate', *ibid.,* Vol. I, 463.
22. J. Hamburger, *Monsieur Littré* (Paris: Flammarion, 1988), 53–4; Jouanna, *op. cit.* (note 14).
23. Littré, *op. cit.* (note 16), Vol. X, 'Dernier coup d'oeil et dernières remarques', xxxvii.
24. Cited are F. C. Maillot, *Traité des fièvres ou irritations cérebro-spinales intermittentes, d'après des observations recueillies en France, en Corse et en Afrique* (Paris: 1836); Roux, *Histoire médicale de l'armée française en Morée pendant la campagne de 1828* (Paris: 1829); W. Twining, *Clinical Illustrations ... of the More Important Diseases of Bengal* (Calcutta: 1835).
25. Littré, *op. cit.* (note 16), Vol. II, 564.
26. Curtin, *Death by Migration* (note 8), admits that the figures may be fuzzy. On the uses of statistics under Napoleon see M.-N. Bourguet, *Déchiffrer la France* (Paris: 1988).
27. D. Larrey, 'Mémoire et observations sur plusieurs maladies qui ont affecté les troupes de l'armée française pendant l'expédition d'Egypte et de Syrie et qui sont endémiques dans ces deux contrées', *Description de l'Egypte, Etat Moderne* (Paris: 1809), Vol. I, 510, 513; R. Desgenettes, *Histoire médicale de l'Armée d'Orient* (Paris: 1830), 12–15, 172–3, 236. S. Jagailoux, *La médîcalisation de l'Egypte au XIXe siècle* (1798–1918) (Paris: 1986).
28. Larrey, *op. cit.* (note 27),
29. N. and J. Dhombres, *Naissance d'un pouvoir: Sciences et savants en France (1793–1824)* (Paris: 1989), 123; C. C. Gillispie, 'Aspects scientifiques de l'expédition d'Egypte (1798–1801)', in H. Laurens (ed.), *L'expédition d'Egypte, 1798–1801* (Paris: 1989), 371–96. Gillispie cautions against anachronistic classification of the memoirs but lists two each in medicine and demography.
30. N. Broc, 'Les explorateurs français du XIXe siècle reconsidérés', *Revue française d'historie d'outre-mer,* lxix (1982), 243; *idem,* 'Les grandes missions scientifiques français au XIXe siècle (Morée, Algérie, Mexique) et leurs travaux géographiques', *Revue d'Histoire des Sciences,* xxxix (1981), 319–58; Laurens, *op. cit.* (note 29), 371; C. C. Gillispie, 'Historical introduction', in C. C. Gillispie and M. Dewachter (eds), *Monuments of Egypt: The Napoleonic Edition* (Princeton: 1987), 5. I include as physicians the seven surgeons and three pharmacists.
31. P. Corsi, *The Age of Lamarck: Evolutionary Theories in France,*

1790–1830 (Berkeley: University of California Press, 1988), 218–29; W. George, 'Bory de Saint-Vincent, Jean Baptiste Georges Marie', *Dictionary of Scientific Biography*, Vol. II, 320–1.

32. N. Broc, 'Les grandes missions scientifiques françaises au XIXe siècle', *Revue d'Histoire des Sciences et de leurs Applications,* xxxiv (1981), 319–58; Lepetit, *op. cit.* (note 3).
33. Bory de Saint-Vincent, *Relation du Voyage* (Paris, 1836), 'Avant-propos', i–iv, 143, 159–60.
34. See, for example, E. W. Said, *Orientalism* (New York: Vintage Books, 1979), 171–6.
35. de St-Vincent, *op. cit.* (note 33), 101–3, 159–60.
36. *Ibid.,* 447–66.
37. 'Exploration scientifique de l'Algérie: Sciences médicales', J. A. N. Périer, *De l'hygiène en Algérie* (Paris: 1847), 2 Vols; I, Ch. 1, 'Acclimatement', 3.
38. *Ibid.,* Vol. I, 28–9.
39. *Ibid.,* 30.
40. On the exploitation of cork oaks near Bône, see D. Prochaska, *Making Algeria French: Colonialism in Bône, 1870–1920* (Cambridge: Cambridge University Press, 1990), 71–7; Périer, *op. cit.* (note 37), Vol. I, 14–15.
41. *Ibid.,* Vol. I, 34.
42. *Ibid.,* 46.
43. *Ibid.,* 56.
44. *Ibid.,* 59–61, quote on 59.
45. *Ibid.,* 66.
46. *Ibid.,* 71.
47. E.-L. Bertherand, *Médecine et hygiène des Arabes* (Paris: G. Baillière, 1855), 561–2; Y. Turin, *Affrontements culturels dans l'Algérie coloniale: Ecoles, médecines, religion, 1830-1880* (Paris: F. Maspero, 1971).
48. J. A. N. Périer, 'Essai sur les croisements ethniques', *Mémoires de la Société d'anthropologie de Paris,* i (1860–3), 69–92, 187–236; ii (1865), 261–374; iii (1868), 211–96.
49. M. Emerit, 'Les methods coloniales de la France sous le Second Empire', *Revue africaine,* xliii (1943), 189, relates a brief flirtation with associationist policy of the period 1858–60. On the consensus see R. R. Betts, *Assimilationism and Association in French Colonial Theory, 1890–1914* (New York: Columbia University Press, 1961); J. J. Cooke, *New French Imperialism, 1880—1910: The Third Republic and Colonial Expansion* (Hamden, Conn.: Archon Books, 1973), 21–2.
50. Great Britain. War Office, *Report of the Causes of Reduced Mortality in the French Army serving in Algeria, Presented to both Houses of Parliament by Command of Her Majesty* (London: 1867), 32.
51. The instrumentalities of medicine within the colonial context are the explicit concern of D. Arnold (ed.), *Imperial Medicine and Indigenous*

Societies (Manchester: Manchester University Press, 1988); *idem, Colonizing the Body: State Medicine and Epidemic Disease in Nineteenth-Century India* (Berkeley: University of California Press, 1993).

5

Disease and Imperialism

Philip D. Curtin

For European doctors in the nineteenth century, tropical medicine and military medicine were nearly synonymous. That connection is one reason why the progress of tropical medicine and the conquest of tropical empire have sometimes been linked – much as imperial conquest of tropical empire has been linked to the flood of new weapons from an industrializing Europe. Both the new weapons and the empirical advances in tropical medicine have been discussed as permissive factors. They may not have caused any particular act of imperial conquest, but they made imperialism cheap in terms of lives and money.[1] No one, to my knowledge, questions the importance of the new weapons, but the role of tropical medicine is less certain.

Figure 1
Mortality of European Troops Serving Overseas: Change Between the 1840s and 1860s

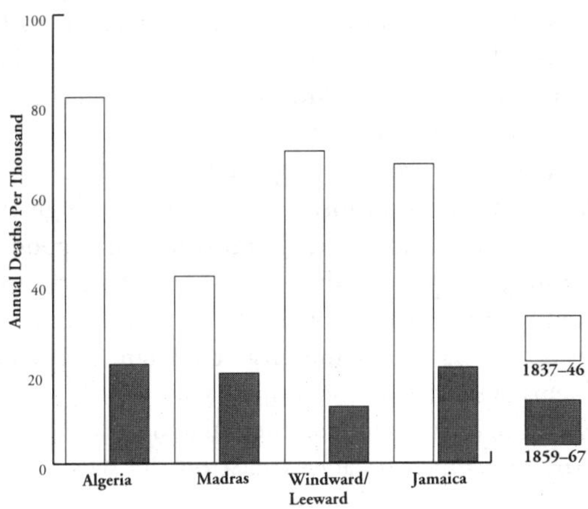

The argument for a causal connection between tropical medicine and imperialism begins with the observation that army doctors in the tropical world made enormous progress in the art of keeping Europeans alive, even before the late-century attention to the role of microbes and mosquitoes. The greatest decrease in tropical death rates for European soldiers came between the 1840s and the 1860s (see Figure 1 and Table 1). The two largest European armies overseas were the French in Algeria and the British in India. Over these two decades, the military death rate in Algeria dropped by 60 per thousand, the military death rate of British troops in India dropped by 22 per thousand, and the change was equally impressive in other tropical territories like the British West Indies or the Dutch East Indies.[2]

Table 1
Military Mortality Change for European Troops Stationed in the Tropics and Sub-Tropics Between the 1840s and 1860s

Years	Algeria	Madras	Windward/Leeward	Jamaica
1837–46	81.54	41.50	69.31	66.44
1859–67	21.93	19.86	12.43	21.15

Annual Average Deaths per Thousand

Source: P. D. Curtin, *Death by Migration,* 36.

The timing is significant. People became conscious of these changes by the late 1860s, and the conventional age of imperialism began with the next decade. But the possible link between imperialism and tropical medicine could be simple accident. European death rates in the tropics decreased, European conquest of the non-Western world increased, but this covariance could be mere coincidence. If a causal link did exist, the direction of the causation remains to be established. The problem is worth a preliminary exploration, looking at some specific successes and failures in tropical medicine and their possible influence on decision making.

The British government's Niger Expedition of 1841–2 is a logical place to begin – an instance of extremely high European mortality before the mid–century transition. If a good medical record encouraged imperial activity in the late century, a bad medical record might well have discouraged it in this earlier period. The Niger Expedition was not a military campaign, but it illustrates some problems of survival in the tropics. The aim was to explore the lower Niger, to open it up for commercial and agricultural development as part of a much broader attack on the slave trade. Three steamers sailed up the Niger with a total of 159 Europeans. The longest time any of the boats spent in the river was just over two months, but even for this brief period the death rate was 350 per thousand, almost all of it from malaria. The malaria morbidity was 82 per cent, and the case-fatality rate was 30 per cent. It would not be statistically legitimate to annualize a death rate of this magnitude, but, if one did, it would have been more than 2,000 per thousand annual strength.[3]

After such a spectacular disaster, the expected response would be withdrawal – like the later French withdrawal from the effort to build a Panama canal before the mosquito vector was known. The Niger disaster was widely publicized. Dickens satirized it in *Bleak House.* But withdrawal is not what happened. The government withdrew the steamers, but it went ahead with a modified extension of the original anti-slave-trade project. The result was more British activity on the West African coast, not less. Without the disaster of the Niger Expedition, the British might have done still more, but within ten years Great Britain had purchased the Danish forts along the Gold Coast and added a new post at Lagos, in spite of public protest and pressure to evacuate the older trading posts and forts.

The Indian Royal Commission of 1863 is a different case in point. It was appointed to enquire into the sanitary state of the army in India. In the background were the high mortality rates from disease in the Crimea, and in India with the suppression of the Rebellion of 1857. What the Commission found was deplorable. The annual mortality of European troops in India over the period 1800–57 had been 69 per thousand, as against 9 per thousand in recent years for troops stationed in England. The commissioners took this difference of 60 per thousand to estimate that it cost £388,000 a year for the additional mortality of keeping an army of that size in India rather than Britain. It continued:

> It is at that expense that we have held dominion there for a century; a company out of every regiment has been sacrificed every 20 months. These companies fade away at the prime of life; leave few children, and have to be replaced, at great cost, by successive shiploads of recruits.[4]

Several alternative solutions were possible. One was to use more Indian troops, but the recent mutiny suggested the danger of that course. Another was to allow more authority to the Native States with their own armies. Still another, less likely, alternative would be to give up all or part of British India. There is no evidence that the

Commission even considered these possibilities. It considered that its task was to find a way to keep the same sized army in India, but with lower troop mortality. As a goal, it set a death rate of ten per thousand for European solders in India, only a little more than the rate then current in Britain itself, and it published a numbered list of 39 separate recommendations to help achieve that end, with a heavy emphasis on barracks design, hospital design and location, ventilation, drainage, clean water, a shift from dry privies to water closets, and disciplined attention to sanitary conditions of all kinds.[5] It was precisely this kind of empirical measure that had produced the striking drop in tropical military mortality elsewhere in the past two decades, and it worked again in this case. In 1869, the mortality rate for all British soldiers in India dropped below 20 per thousand. In 1907, with the new knowledge of germ theory and the mosquito vector, it dropped below ten.

The causal direction of this case seems clear. In 1863, the commissioners wanted empire on the cheap; they therefore set out to improve the health of the army in the tropics. It is possible, nevertheless, that their success encouraged still more imperial ventures at some later time.

These medical reforms were part of a wider set of post-Mutiny military reforms, beginning with the Indian Army in the early 1860s and extending to the British army at home over the next decade or so. The British phase of these reforms came to be known as the Cardwell reforms, after Edward Cardwell, Secretary of State for War in the Gladstone government of 1868–74. The Indian and domestic military reforms gave the British military, in the Indian army and at home, a new confidence and a desire to try out the new weapons, tactics and organization in a field situation. This underlying hope to conduct manoeuvres with live ammunition was in the background of two remarkable expeditions in Africa – the invasion of Ethiopia with the march to Magdala by the Indian Army in 1868 and the invasion of Asante and the march to Kumasi in 1874.

Both had a chosen objective – a particular place to capture and destroy. In both, the army evacuated its expeditionary force within six months, leaving behind no political or strategic changes worth mentioning. The real value of these expeditions in retrospect was the practice they gave the younger officers, new lessons in strategy and tactics for the high command, and the demonstration of what British armies could do to the Queen's enemies. In that era of racism and imperialism, the demonstrations of power 'to maintain white man's prestige' were serious objectives for the military and political theorists. Contemporaries hailed both expeditions as marvels of military and tropical medicine. Because of these claims, the two expeditions illustrate some of the relationships between tropical medicine and imperialism.

As a problem for tropical medicine, the Magdala Expedition should have been a cinch. The troops, armed with the new breech-loading Snider rifles, landed on a desert coast and marched immediately into the highlands. No cholera, no malaria, no yellow fever; and enteric fever was negligible. The expedition fought only two engagements, with no-one killed in action and only a few wounded. The military medical report on the expedition was full of self-congratulation. A leader in *The Times* at the end of the expedition said, among other things:

> A few wounds on our side against a great slaughter on the other duly represents the difference between civilized and semi-barbarous warriors.... Certainly, we are all aware that without science it would be impossible to overcome the peculiar difficulties of the Expedition.[6]

This opinion was virtually unchallenged at the time or in retrospect, and it illustrates a significant point about nineteenth-century thought on the subject of military death. Death from enemy action was part of the 'fortunes of war', which brave men risked when they went into battle. Death from disease was more ordinary, less honourable and often unreported. In fact, European soldiers on the Magdala Expedition died from disease at an annualized rate of 34 per thousand, against the annual average for troops in Britain of 8 per thousand. Instead of the 'few wounds' of *The Times* leader, the expedition cost the lives of 107 British soldiers and 181 Indian soldiers who would not have died if they had stayed at home. These numbers are not large, but they count for something in a campaign whose sole achievement was to rescue 67 hostages held by the Emperor Tewodros of Ethiopia.

The British press said very little about these deaths, and next to nothing about the death of Indian civilians who took part. For the march to Magdala, the British official reports indicate that 41,000 civilian 'followers' landed on the African coast – mainly from India, but a few from China and elsewhere. Of these, only 24,000 re-embarked for the voyage back to Bombay. The remaining 17,000, 40 per cent of the total, either died or deserted in Africa.[7] Most of them apparently died from malnutrition, lack of medical care and lack of provision for evacuating their sick. The lack of publicity for these deaths illustrates still another nineteenth-century peculiarity in evaluating death. British soldiers counted most; 'native troops' like those of the Indian army counted less; a civilian non-British labour force hardly counted at all.

The lessons drawn from the Magdala campaign were important because it was so widely publicized at the time. It was prominently investigated by a Select Committee of the House of Commons, mainly because it had cost £9 million, when the original estimate had been £2 million. Aside from a few complaints about the flogging of muleteers, the Indian side of the expedition was hardly mentioned, and the Indian loss of life was simply ignored. Then, and in retrospect, the Magdala campaign was regarded as a model of brilliant organization and a lesson that war in Tropical Africa was possible with minimal loss.[8] Whatever the reality, the claimed achievements of military medicine certainly did suggest that future imperial adventures would be equally cheap.

The Asante Expedition of 1874 was a similar campaign to exercise the troops, but in a different theatre and with a different outcome. The West African forest belt had a reputation as the 'white man's grave' going back centuries,[9] topped off by the recent Niger Expedition and other horrors. The British kept their posts there in spite of the cost, though other Europeans did not. The Danes sold theirs in 1851, the French evacuated theirs in 1871, and the Dutch sold their Gold Coast forts to Britain in 1872. Even the British made a tentative decision to withdraw and then thought better of it.

Meanwhile, in the War Office, the Cardwell reforms had taken place, with a new form of military medical organization more independent of regimental controls. Cardwell had brought Garnet Wolseley into the War Office to help build a more professional officer corps. Wolseley and others were anxious to show what the professionalized army could do, egged on by intra-service rivalries with the Indian Army crowd that had pulled off the Magdala triumph, and by a desire to prove that European troops could fight well in the humid tropics.

The opportunity came in 1873, when an Asante army invaded the hinterland of Cape Coast Castle on the Gold Coast. The Colonial Office was not anxious for a major encounter, but Wolseley was, and he got his way, with planning support from Surgeon-General Sir William Muir, the head of the Army Medical Department. Lord Derby hailed the expedition in advance as 'an engineer's war, a doctor's war'. The plans called for a demonstration campaign at the height of the dry season in January and February 1874. They included meticulous preparation for the march inland, keeping the bulk of the army on ships offshore, safe from fevers, and drinking distilled sea water until the last moment. A quarter of the officers were medical officers. The bulk of the troops were on the shore less than two months. They advanced the 140 miles to the Asante capital at Kumasi and burned it before hurrying back to the ships.

The medical achievement was impressive. Loss from disease alone was limited to just over 17 per thousand – against 26 per thousand on the Magdala campaign and 151 per thousand annually for British troops in barracks in West Africa in the immediate past.[10] Forty per cent of the deaths from disease were from malaria and 28 per cent from gastro-intestinal infections. The latter was a major improvement over the Magdala experience, where 75 per cent of the deaths from disease had been gastro-intestinal,[11] and the change was based on a real improvement in army hygiene. For Magdala the troops used sand and charcoal filters incapable of affecting bacteria. Similar filters were also issued for the march to Kumasi, but the new recommendations included boiled drinking water treated with potassium permanganate as well.[12]

The public reaction in Europe was immediate and favourable. Seven first-hand book-length accounts were published before the end of 1874, and the expedition was thoroughly covered in the newspaper press, including the medical press. Again the medical achievement was vastly exaggerated. Lord Carnarvon at the Colonial Office claimed that the death rate, which he gave as 23 per thousand, was about the same as the death-rate in Britain,[13] but he compared it to the British rate for population of all ages over a whole year, not a mere two months for a population at risk who were in the prime of life and peak physical condition. The contemporaneous death-rate from disease alone for British troops in Britain was an annual average of less than 8 per thousand. The annualized loss from the disease on the Asante Expedition would have been 102 per thousand.[14]

Specialists in military and tropical medicine should have recognized the fraud, but their main reaction was to accept the expedition as evidence that European troops could be used anywhere in the world without exceptional losses from disease.[15] Continental medical authorities accepted the same claims.[16] The achievement was to be cited again and again throughout the rest of the century as evidence of the low risk of disease in the humid tropics. And the timing, just before the European scramble for Africa began, suggests that it influenced what followed.

But, like the Madgala claims, some accounts of the Asante Expedition were bogus and even the true reports created a wrong impression. The march on Kumasi was a lucky fluke; no other campaign of equivalent size anywhere in tropical Africa over the next 20 years equalled the disease record of that expedition. Part of its success was based on the unusual practice of giving medical officers real authority over the plans. Part was the choice of a short campaign in two dry-season months, an option seldom available in wartime. Part was luck, including a very narrow escape from a yellow-fever epidemic. Tropical medicine could not yet achieve what some claimed for that campaign. In 1895, after the germ theory was well known, impure water could be identified, the French sent an expeditionary force to conquer Madagascar, with the Asante campaign as the explicit example of what to expect from disease. That expedition lost a third of its men from disease alone in less than six months.

The sum of these four cases may do more to illustrate the complexity of the problem than it does to demonstrate that tropical medicine caused imperialism, or the reverse. The losses of the Niger Expedition may have slowed the rate of growth in imperial activity, but that was all. The heavy losses in India over the first half of the century led to medical reforms – not less imperialism – though the success of the reforms may have made later imperialism cheaper. The Magdala and Asante campaigns supported the belief that tropical warfare was now affordable, but that conclusion was wrong. It was not simply that tropical medicine cleared the way for imperialism. The new public health measures helped, but the genuine improvement was equalled and sometimes outweighed by misunderstanding downright misrepresentation.

Notes

1. Daniel R. Headrick, *The Tools of Empire: Technology and European Imperialism in the Nineteenth Century* (Oxford & New York: Oxford University Press, 1981). I have argued this case myself in P. D. Curtin *et al., African History* (London: Longman, 1978), 445–8.
2. P. D. Curtin, *Death by Migration: Europe's Encounter with the Tropical World in the Nineteenth Century* (Cambridge & New York: Cambridge University Press, 1989), 36, 194–5, 199–202.
3. P. D. Curtin, *The Image of Africa: British Ideas and Action, 1780–1850* (Madison: University of Wisconsin, 1964), 486–7.
4. Report of the Commissioners, *Parliamentary Papers* (hereafter *PP*), 1863, xix (C.3184), xi.
5. Report of the Commissioners, *PP,* 1863, xix (C.3184), lxxxii.
6. *The Times,* 1 May, 1868, 6.
7. *PP,* 1868–9, vi, 142–3.
8. For retrospective views see Gustave A. Reynaud, *Considerations*

sanitaires sur l'expédition de Madagascar et quelques autres expéditions coloniales, françaises et anglaises (Paris: 1898), 34–5; John William Fortescue, *A History of the British Army* (13 vols, London: Macmillan, 1930), xiii, 474.

9. P. D. Curtin, 'The White Man's Grave: Image and reality, 1780–1850', *Journal of British Studies,* (1961), 94–110.
10. *Idem,* 'The end of the "White Man's Grave": Nineteenth-century mortality in West Africa', *Journal of Interdisciplinary History,* xxi (1990), 71.
11. Anthony D. Home, 'Medical History of the war in the Gold Coast Protectorate in 1873', Great Britain, *Army Medical Service Report* (*AMSR*) (1868), 205–8. Richard Eustace to Sir Alexander Armstrong, 26 August, 1873, *PP,* 1874, xlvii (C.891), 98–9.
12. *Ibid.;* Home, *op. cit.* (note 11), 223.
13. Quoted in W. Walton Claridge, *A History of the Gold Coast and Ashanti,* (2 vols, London: Cass, 1964, first published 1915), ii, 166.
14. That is, the annual average mortality for the period 1869–77 (Curtin, *op. cit.* (note 2), Table A4, 168).
15. *Medical Times and Gazette,* 18 February, 1874. See also *Lancet,* 21 March, 1874, i, 421; *Medical Times and Gazette,* 14 March, 1874, 293; *Lancet,* 10 June, 1874, i, 889.
16. Léon Colin, 'L'expédition anglaise de la côte d'or: Etude d'hygiène militarie et de géographie médicale', *Annales d'hygiène et de médecine coloniale,* xi (2nd series), 37–40, 52–4; E. Rochefort, 'Etude médicale sur l'expédition anglaise contre les ashantis', *Archives de médecine navale,* xxi (1874), 321–46.

6

Tropical Medicine in Nineteenth-Century Brazil: The Case of the 'Escola Tropicalista Bahiana', 1860–1890

Julyan G. Peard

One of the remarkable aspects about the growing interest in the history of tropical medicine of the last ten years has been the relative absence of Latin America from the story. The bulk of the research concerns Africa, India and other parts of the European colonial empires. Indeed, the terms 'tropical medicine' and 'colonial medicine' are sometimes used interchangeably because it is assumed that tropical medicine was developed almost exclusively by Europeans – joined later by North Americans – due to the demands of empire, demands that quickened just as the germ theory of disease gained acceptance and provided one of the most successful paradigms for understanding tropical disorders.[1] The omission of Latin America is regrettable because it boasts the oldest tradition of Western medicine in the Americas, a tradition that stretches back, in some cases, to early colonial times when the Spaniards set up the first universities in the hemisphere.[2] In some Latin American countries medical study came later. In Brazil, for example, the first medical schools were founded as late as 1808 and they only became degree-granting institutions in the 1830s. But whether a country traced its medical teaching heritage back to the colonial era or to the national era, it was certainly the case that in the second half of the nineteenth century all of the largest Latin American nations trained their doctors locally and followed a Western European tradition of medical education. Moreover, because most of these countries lay within what was then called the 'torrid zone', Latin American medical communities and the diseases the doctors wrote about would seem to be an obvious source of interest for medical historians and social historians interested in the rise of tropical medicine.[3]

One of the reasons that historians have neglected Latin America in relation to the rise of tropical medicine is that, until recently, tropical medicine was studied in relation to the stages of widening European concern regarding colonial health and, as Arnold has pointed out, the dynamics of the encounter between European and indigenous society was little considered.[4] In the Latin American case there was, possibly, even less interest because its dominant intellectual traditions were seen as no more than extensions of the metropolitan ones. The argument was often made that nineteenth-century medicine in Latin America was purely imitative of European, particularly French, medicine and, that it was only when the Europeans turned to tropical medicine and began to make a series of spectacular breakthroughs that a few Latin American doctors, trained in the new centres for tropical medicine in Europe and the United States, became active contributors to Western medicine. Older medical histories of Latin America told stories to gauge how far Western medicine had been adopted. The more critical or pessimistic authors decried the fact that Latin Americans did not imitate the advances of European medical science more closely and thus emerge from their backwardness. The more optimistic authors pointed to successful episodes of medical discovery in Latin America in order to show that the area was less backward than was generally assumed.[5] Neither explored the possibility of relatively independent strands in the tradition of Latin American medicine.

While it is true that much Latin American medicine was imitative of Europe, there are good reasons for historians to re-examine the record of Latin American doctors, especially for the era before Mansonian tropical medicine. Firstly, one reason is simply that this is perhaps the most neglected period in the history of medicine in nineteenth-century Latin America and much remains nebulous. Thus individual doctors are catapulted as heroes into the history of medicine at the turn of the century but we have little sense of whether they represent continuity with a tradition or a break with it. Secondly, in Latin America European medicine made the transition from maritime to territorial empire very early on in the history of Western expansionism.[6] Thus the problem of manipulating tropical disease environments was an old one. It is safe to assume that some of the issues that confronted the European colonial powers at the end of the nineteenth century had been faced earlier in Latin America. The long-term health of Europeans in the tropics, the health and calibre of a tropical labour force, the specificity of the diseases of warm climates, were all questions of long standing in Latin America. A study of the tradition of Western medicine in Latin America can, therefore, provide a more complete picture of Western medicine overall and the diverse ways in which it was taken up in regions linked to, yet far from, metropolitan sources. Thirdly, the nineteenth-century movements for independence in Latin America presented leaders with the challenge of constituting new nations within tropical environments. As Benedict Anderson has argued, this meant more than the staking out of boundaries and the setting up of stable governments. It meant, too, the creation of 'imagined' communities wherein the meanings of the nation were articulated, and the bonds tying together different groups and individuals spelled out. Literature, religion, science and medicine all played crucial roles in the creation of this imagined national community.[7] Given this, we may ask, were there no pre-Mansonian attempts to create a medicine more relevant to the conditions and problems of the new tropical nations and to resist a passive imitation of the agenda of temperate European medicine?

My research on nineteenth-century Brazil suggests that assumptions about the blanket passivity of all Latin American physicians are simplistic and that there was a search for a distinctive medicine of the 'torrid zone'. This search tends to be forgotten as historians focus on tropical medicine and its relationship to European colonies, United States' imperialism, and the rise of the germ theory. Specifically, my research is on a group of doctors in Salvador da Bahia, Brazil, who formed what came to be known as the 'Bahian Tropicalista School' and who practised in the latter half of the nineteenth century. These doctors were clearly groping for an original approach to medicine in their tropical country while, at the same time, anxiously seeking approval from the European medical community to legitimate their endeavours. In this article I view their work on beriberi and hookworm as examples of a growing trend in nineteenth-century Brazil to see the diseases of warm climates as somehow distinct from those of temperate Europe, and suggest that Brazilian doctors were better equipped than Europeans to wax eloquent about these disorders.[8] I argue that the Tropicalistas were part of a generation that attempted to define this distinction and to focus on the importance of the tropics in medicine for national, and not colonial, reasons; that they were also part of a generation of doctors which straddled the two paradigms of disease most prominent in the second half of the nineteenth century, the environmentalist and the new germ theory; that far from being passive doctors, they kept very much abreast of new developments in European medicine drawing upon them selectively and creatively; and, that, although practising in regions far from Europe, they were linked to an international network made up of doctors either currently working in tropical regions, or of doctors who had previously worked in these regions, but had then returned to Europe. I focus first on the social and historical setting of the Tropicalistas, and then on their discoveries and research into beriberi and hookworm in Brazil.

Social and Historical Setting

Independent since 1822, it was in the second half of the nineteenth century, and particularly from the 1870s onwards, that Brazil came to define its contours as a nation. Brazil's humiliating near defeat in the Paraguayan War (1865–70) led to a deep self-questioning by the Brazilian élite about the obstacles to the nation's progress.[9] Moreover, the country's shift to modernization as evidenced in the growth of an urban culture confronting the old rural and aristocratic one, in the rise of positivism, evolutionary ideas and republicanism, in the beginning of European immigration, and the stimulus of new wealth, all led to a profound critique of Brazilian society, especially a questioning of the axis institutions in imperial Brazil, slavery and monarchy.[10] Foremost among the critics were the urban middle classes, strongly influenced by positivism, many of whose ideas were forged in the schools of law, engineering and medicine located in cities around Brazil. As the only institutions of higher education in the country, the degrees earned at these schools conferred more than a means of entry into a specific profession. They also supplied a stepping-stone from which ambitious young men entered politics and the civil service. The most successful of doctors, for example, defined the medical profession as one concerned as much with the problems of society as with the needs of the sick. Their opinions carried a good deal of weight. They held important political and administrative posts at state and national levels. The wide range of their concerns is well illustrated by the work and interests of the doctors who made up the Bahian Topicalista School of Medicine.[11]

The Bahian Tropicalista School of Medicine, active between 1865 and 1890, an informal 'school' formed by about 30 Brazilian, and a handful of foreign, physicians, made new discoveries in parasitology, contributed to ongoing debates on beriberi, parasitology, leprosy, tuberculosis, dracontiasis, and helped reformulate the then-accepted pattern of Brazilian nosology. The Tropicalistas started as an outsider movement critiquing the Brazilian medical schools for their outdated teaching methods and curriculam. Above all, they criticized Brazilian doctors for their lack of original investigation into the disorders of Brazil.[12]

The three founding members of the Tropicalista school were

foreigners who made Brazil their home. Otto Wucherer (1820–75), arguably the most important member of the group, was born of German parents in Portugal and moved to Brazil as a young boy. He returned to Europe for his medical training and graduated from the University of Tubingen in 1841 at a time when Germany was beginning to play a leading role in laboratory medicine.[13] He then spent time as a medical assistant at St Bartholomew's Hospital in London and, after a brief stint in Portugal, returned to Brazil in 1843, becoming in 1847 physician to the German community in Salvador, Bahia. He was one of the founders of the Tropicalista journal, *Gazeta Médica da Bahia,* to which he contributed a handful of seminal articles based on original research which became crucial to the identity of the Tropicalistas.[14] His best-known work was in the field of parasitology: in 1865 he isolated hookworm parasites for the first time in Brazil, and he was the first person to isolate the embryonic filaria.[15]

A second important founding figure of the Tropicalista school was John L. Paterson (1820–82). A Scotsman, he graduated from the University of Aberdeen in 1841 and travelled to Brazil in his early twenties encouraged by his older brother, Alexander, who had set up a practice with the British community in Salvador. John succeeded unexpectedly to this practice in 1843 when his brother died suddenly. Paterson spent most of the rest of his life as a doctor in Brazil although he made several extended visits to England and Scotland. During these visits, he frequented the most advanced hospitals in Britain, and attended the lectures of prominent physicians. In 1869 he worked with Joseph Lister in Edinburgh. This was a turning point in his life and he was rapidly won over to Lister's method of antisepsis, and later introduced some younger Bahian physicians, on European medical tours, to Lister and his practices. In 1865 Paterson proposed to a handful of his associates in Bahia that informal meetings be held in order to exchange ideas, discuss cases, and keep up with developments in medicine and surgery. These meetings, held on a fortnightly basis, eventually led to the birth of the Tropicalista school. At the meetings, where there were earnest discussions on the work in parasitology of Angelo Dubini, Theodor Bilharz and Wilhelm Griesinger, among others, Wucherer was encouraged to continue his own research.

From these discussions, too, came the idea of starting a medical journal, an idea staunchly supported by the third in the triad of founding members of the Tropicalista school, Jose Francisco da Silva Lima (1826–1910). Born in Portugal, Silva Lima was 14 when he moved with his parents to Salvador where his father became a merchant. He graduated from the Medical School in Bahia in 1851. Between 1853 and 1881 he made five trips to Europe to advance his medical knowledge. If Wucherer provided the impetus for the original research on which other Tropicalistas could build, it was Silva Lima who provided the perseverance and continuity which led to the group's success. A long-time editor of the *Gazeta Médica da Bahia,* he contributed some 200 articles to the journal.

As foreigners these men were excluded from the existing network of patronage so crucial for the advancement of medical careers in nineteenth-century Brazil. None of them, for example, ever taught at the Bahia Medical School, the most prestigious medical institution in the city. In spite of this they attracted a core of supporters especially among younger doctors, students and political progressives. The success of the early Tropicalistas in winning adherents cannot simply be explained by the fact that they were resourceful and ambitious, or that European medicine was beginning to make path-breaking strides. These factors were crucial, but they were not enough to explain the rise of the Tropicalistas as the most successful research-oriented doctors in nineteenth-century Brazil. In the course of the century there had been other notable foreign doctors working in Brazil and many Brazilian doctors eager for more scientific approaches to medicine. But they had never resulted in a movement such as the Tropicalista.[16]

What enabled the Tropicalistas to attract a following and initiate a movement for change within Brazilian medicine was that their criticism of the *status quo* in the medical establishment, their striving for innovation, their doctrines of 'progress' and 'science', all dovetailed with a broader political agenda for change which, from the 1870s onwards was slowly being defined within pockets of discontent all over the Brazilian Empire. The Tropicalistas argued that Brazilians had an important contribution to make to the international patrimony of medicine by developing an expertise on disease in the tropics. They held that, just as doctors in Europe were unravelling the mysteries of the disorders that surrounded them, so they were part of a new generation of doctors in Brazil who must seek to understand, control, and manipulate the pathologies of the tropics. In order to investigate these tropical disorders they made full use of the research arsenal of European medicine such as, for example, medical statistics, new clinical methods based on measurement and applied physiology, the use of chemistry in analysing body fluids, increased understanding of haematology and, above all, microscopy which they pioneered in

Bahia.[17] For their work they received no official institutional support or funding. Yet, in spite of this, they were successful in forming an institutional framework from which they became an important innovating force in Bahian, and ultimately Brazilian, medicine.

Two institutions were central to their success. One was the Santa Casa de Misericordia charity hospital, and the other was their journal, the *Gazeta Médica da Bahia.* In the Santa Casa hospital, which attended mainly to the poor of the city and its outskirts and to sailors, the Tropicalistas found a niche for themselves.[18] Here, interested students observed and assisted many of their cases, some of whom received their only practical instruction in the use of the microscope or in the art of autopsy from the Tropicalistas. The Santa Casa also became a means of centralizing the otherwise isolated inquiries of the Tropicalistas, and a place where like-minded doctors could experiment with new surgical methods and therapies which they either read about in the European and North American medical literature, or, at times, acquired from local healers.[19]

The second institution crucial to the success of the Tropicalistas was the journal they founded in 1866. An analysis of the journal provides fascinating insights into the several aims of the Tropicalistas, aims which sometimes pulled them in opposing directions. On the one hand, the journal followed a hallowed attempt to reproduce Western medicine in the tropics. Thus, through the journal the Tropicalistas wanted to forge a strong, well-informed medical profession in Bahia, drawing from a common pool of scientific knowledge. They also used the journal to advocate an alliance between doctors and pharmacists against folk healers and quacks; to promote a closing of ranks among doctors, thereby keeping physicians' disputes away from public scrutiny; and to propose ideas, new for Brazil, on the importance to the medical community of creating a submissive patient who recognized the absolute authority of the physician.[20] On the other hand, the journal was founded in order to stake out a medically distinctive field for Brazilian doctors. It is this aspect of the journal which is of most interest to the historian of early tropical medicine and it is this aspect of the journal that the Tropicalistas saw as paramount. The journal was to be a forum for the findings of doctors working in Brazil. As an editorial in the *Gazeta Médica da Bahia* put it: 'We always prefer to [report] on our own investigations than to transcribe articles on foreign medicine because our main objective is to clarify and develop the study of Brazilian medicine.'[21]

It was this objective that led them to ask questions which were at the heart of tropical medicine at the turn of the century: Was there a geography of disease with specific illnesses confined to tropical regions? Did heat and moisture favour the multiplication of harmful micro-organisms thus making tropical regions particularly disease ridden? Did tropical climate *per se* have a deleterious influence upon human beings, regardless of whether persons lived within a milieu of good sanitation, followed a sound diet and a regimen of healthy exercise? Did tropical climate affect various races differently? Was acclimatization possible for whites? Could Brazilians be healthy?

The answers to these questions were not merely of medical interest. They were central to establishing whether it was possible for Brazil to view itself as a 'civilized' nation in the tropics. For Brazilian doctors, such as the Tropicalistas, the production of a national 'brazilianized' medicine was a way of contesting the Europeans' notion that the tropics were inherently unhealthy, degenerating, and alien to European culture.[22] Such stereotypes not only left doctors practising in the tropics bereft of real agency (since the climate, topography and racial genealogies seemed impossible to eradicate), but they also dimmed the hopes of the new Latin American élites to transform their countries into healthy and progressive nations, accepted as equals by the leading European nations. Doctors, like the Brazilian Tropicalistas, were of central importance in promoting the idea of a progressive Brazilian nation because they could make recommendations for improving the health of all classes of Brazilians and, more crucially, because they provided conceptual tools whereby the national intelligentsia could resist derogatory labels of difference and inferiority produced by European scientific and medical discourse. When the Tropicalistas argued that understanding the disorders of Brazil was really no different from understanding the disorders of temperate Europe, they appealed to those members of the Brazilian élite struggling to assert that, although Brazilians were racially mixed and natives of the tropics, this made them merely different from Europeans, neither better nor worse.

The Evolution of a Tropicalista Agenda: Beriberi

One of the key disorders which came to define the Tropicalistas was beriberi. In 1866 Jose Francisco da Silva Lima warned of an epidemic outbreak of beriberi in the city of Bahia in an article published in the *Gazeta Médica da Bahia*.[23] Between 1863 and 1866 Silva Lima attended 32 patients who presented such similar symptoms of weakness, numbness in the extremities, oedema, degeneration of muscular tissue and, in some cases, paralysis, that he strongly suspected that he was dealing with a specific disorder. As he made enquiries among his colleagues he found that they too had recently treated similar cases. In discussing the cases with his close friend and colleague, Dr Paterson, the latter directed Silva Lima to a reference in Dr Copland's *Medical Dictionary* which described a disorder known in India as *barbiers* or *beriberi.* To Silva Lima the description sounded remarkably like what he had been treating. In subsequent reading, Silva Lima became convinced he was dealing with beriberi, a conclusion further validated for him by his correspondence with a French naval physician and expert on beriberi, A. Le Roy de Mericourt.[24] As a result of Silva Lima's 'discovery' of beriberi in Bahia, an editorial in the *Gazeta Médica* of November 1866 warned other doctors of the danger of this new illness reaching 'epidemic' proportions in the state of Bahia.[25]

It is instructive to look at Silva Lima's attempts to decipher the question of the aetiology of beriberi in order to get a sense of his place within contemporary ideas of epidemic disease in the tropics. He held the disorder to be a blood intoxication caused by miasma in the tropics. Miasma, a common theme in Western medicine, believed to emanate from filth, stagnant water, churned-up soil, rotting vegetation, was held to be particularly lethal when found in the tropics.[26] It seemed clear to Silva Lima that the blood intoxication which he believed led to beriberi, was caused by some agent which relied for its existence on the climatic conditions of the tropics. But he was aware that the concept of tropical miasma was so general as to be almost irrelevant in the explanation of disease aetiology:

> The great kingdom of tropical disorders, ... [which lies] to the north and south of the equator contains a large number of disorders peculiar to these regions .... Unfortunately, here as in ... the rest of the regions within the tropical zone, we only know that climatic conditions favour this or that tropical disorder, without knowing the actual cause of these disorders.[27]

As a pragmatic physician working in the tropics, Silva Lima wanted to go beyond the blanket term of 'tropical miasma' to search for causes. Working within long-established European aetiological traditions of topography and climate, Silva Lima attempted to tease out which might be the most dangerous topographical and climatic conjunctures for those who were predisposed to the disorder. There was little novelty in the conclusions he reached. For example, he considered sudden climatic changes to be an important contributing factor. Even more dangerous were long periods of heat combined with humidity and unhygienic conditions. An individual's constitution weakened as a result of former illness, or of a life of vice and debauchery, increased the chances of contracting the disorder, as did pregnancy in the case of women. He believed that hygienic conditions were crucially important. Silva Lima was not wholly satisfied with these explanations, however, and for the next two decades he continued to mull over the possible causes of beriberi. Attuned to the debates of his time, he was willing to consider the possibility of a narrower and more specific cause. For example, he was intrigued by the diet deficiency theory proposed in connection with the Dutch East Indies and the Japanese navy, but he was unable to reconcile this theory with the fact that people with apparently good diets were known to have succumbed to the disease.[28] In the end he continued to adhere to the broader miasmatic/environmentalist explanations, professing that 'for the moment most of the evidence supports the miasmatic theory'.[29]

Silva Lima's writings on beriberi show him to be a doctor well within the European medical tradition. But he also represented a spirit of reform in Brazilian medicine. He was willing to challenge European doctors by questioning accepted geographical frontiers for a disorder such as beriberi, long held not to be found in Brazil. He stressed the importance of Brazilian doctors using their own clinical practice as the prime source for the discovery of illnesses of warm climates and, although he accepted that a tropical climate was the fundamental context for beriberi outbreaks, he wanted to investigate exactly how a tropical climate was relevant to the disorder. His position was not unlike those European sanitarians who were aware that, although filth was the context of many diseases, it did not adequately explain them.

It was Silva Lima's younger colleague, Antonio Pacifico Pereira (1846–1922), another key figure among the Tropicalistas, who took up the challenge of further unravelling the puzzle of beriberi. In the end, however, he too fell back upon environmentalist explanations. Indeed, the Tropicalistas' juggling of concepts from a waning paradigm in European medicine with that of a nascent one, and their tendency to straddle the older miasmatic/environmentalist approach with the newer parasitical/bacteriological one, is particularly well illustrated in the work of Pacifico Pereira. In 1879–80 Pacifico Pereira carried out original research on beriberi focusing on the pathological anatomy of the disorder and, in particular, the haemotological alterations in the blood of beriberi patients.[30] He performed autopsies on over 60 beriberi victims, making detailed examinations of their diseased tissues, blood and urine. From his reading on beriberi, his clinical observations and his autopsies, Pereira arrived at the conclusion that the cause of beriberi was 'anoxemia' or lack of oxygen in the blood. What then caused anoxemia? The common denominator Pereira found in all his reading and in his own clinical experience was the tropical climate: '[I]t seems irrefutable that ... beriberi is a disorder of the tropical zone, and especially of hot and damp areas.'[31] Like Silva Lima, however, Pereira sought to probe exactly how the damp and heat affected a person. For an answer he turned to the German physician and hygienist, Max von Pettenkofer. Quoting from the latter, Pereira held that it was crucial for the regeneration of the body's tissues that a process of oxygenation occur. By this he meant the supply of plentiful oxygen to the blood which, as it circulated through the tissues of the body, performed a purifying process.[32] The problem with a hot, damp climate according to Pereira, was that it inhibited the process of oxygenation so that, as the blood was deprived of oxygen, it was unable to wholly throw off the poisons of the body and carry out a thorough regeneration of the tissues. An extreme form of this condition caused anoxemia which, he believed, led to beriberi.[33]

In subsequent writings Pereira ignored the climatic fatalism inherent in his theory. Instead he became increasingly preoccupied with what practical steps should be taken to neutralize the dangers of poor oxygenation in the tropics. Believing that exercise could increase the process of oxygenation of the blood, he argued that schools should not merely be places to instil intellectual and moral ideas but places where the physical aspect of students should be developed and the deleterious effects of the tropics reversed: 'Physiology clearly shows us that *air and exercise are even more necessary to physical development in a tropical climate* because it is an incontestable fact that the organism lacks an abundant provision of oxygen for respiration and nutrition.'[34]

Pereira's practical recommendations for schools to combat the drawbacks of what he termed a 'debilitating' climate and a 'decadent' race included specifications on the spatial layout in schools in order to ensure a good circulation of the air, a reformed programme of activities, and a re-scheduling of students' time to make periods of passive learning briefer. As an extension of his medical activities, Pacifico Pereira became an active school reformer whose work became so well-known in Brazil that he was an important participant in the loud and contentious national debate over the reform of imperial education culminating in the 1884 Saboia Law.[35]

Pereira's work was not entirely within the old environmentalist paradigm of disease. Influenced by the path-breaking discoveries then being made in Western medicine, he was also interested in exploring the possible bacteriological cause of beriberi. In his investigation of the pathological anatomy of beriberi he reported that he had found a particular micro-organism in the blood of almost all the beriberi patients he had examined.[36] Despite this finding, Pereira resisted concluding that the micro-organisms were the cause of the disease. The micro-organisms, he explained, also existed in the blood of patients suffering from other disorders. Moreover, although he was able to cultivate them according to Pasteur's methods, he had not been able to generate the disease in laboratory animals. Pereira's caution in this area of his research can be attributed to the simple fact that as a good scientist he recognized that he had not proved the bacterial cause of beriberi (and we know he was right to conclude this). Nevertheless, it is arguable that his caution cannot be ascribed simply to his excellence as a scientist. Pereira had less 'evidence' for his theory of anoxemia than he had for the possible bacteriological link to beriberi. By 1883 he had examined the blood of some 100 patients and, according to his reports, consistently found the same micro-organism.[37] Indeed, a physician from Rio de Janeiro who turned up the same finding did make the link and had his findings splashed across the news headlines – much to Pereira's annoyance.[38]

Even though Pereira himself never pursued further research along the lines of bacteriology, he proposed a way in which both the micro-organism and environmentalist factors might be harmonized in the aetiology of beriberi. He hypothesized that the process of anoxemia, for him the main cause of beriberi, created the conditions in the blood of the victim for micro-organisms to carry out their harmful effects.[39] In other words, by proposing that a micro-organism was only able to become pathological in combination with a certain environment, and by giving primary aetiological weight to that environment, Pereira sought a balance between two approaches to disease aetiology.[40] He encouraged his younger colleague, A. Pacheco Mendes, to continue the investigation along these lines.[41] Pereira himself felt far more comfortable with the older theories of environment, and the transformative powers of hygiene and sanitation upon a malleable population, theories which had pushed him to become an active and visible member of the Bahia community. In this case, Pereira was on the cusp of a conceptual shift in tropical medicine from a generalized notion of disease dependent upon many ambiguous variables, to a search for specific causes and treatments in each particular disease.[42] As a physician working in a tropical environment, stereotyped by Europeans as inherently unhealthy, Pereira's fundamental concern was to show that sanitary changes and progressive social policies could effectively address the problem of achieving a healthy population in a tropical milieu. He had spent many years translating this concern into practice and, although we know that ultimately bacteriology did much to remove the stigma of 'tropicality' from Brazil, Pereira continued to perform the task primarily as a sanitarian and social reformer in a tropical environment.

The Evolution of a Tropicalista Agenda: Hookworm

Hookworm was another of the disorders which became central to the identity and research agenda of the Tropicalistas. The case of hookworm illustrates even more clearly than beriberi the pull in opposite directions of the Tropicalistas as they contributed to the new parasitological theories of disease but continued to find the environmental paradigm a powerful tool with which to confront health in the tropics and to frame their demands for improved social conditions.

In December 1865 Dr Otto Wucherer was called to the monastery of San Bento to attend to Delfino, a slave belonging to a plantation in Santo Amaro. Wucherer diagnosed the patient as suffering from an extreme case of what Brazilian doctors then termed 'hypoemia tropical' or 'cansanço' which, shortly thereafter, caused the patient's death.[43] An autopsy revealed numerous worms in the victim's small intestine which Wucherer identified as 'anckylostoma duodenale'.[44] By mid-1866 Wucherer had performed another six autopsies, all of which revealed large clusters of the parasite. The *Gazeta Médica* hailed the finding as an important breakthrough. It stated that Wucherer had demonstrated that slaves and agricultural workers, the main victims of the disorder, suffered from anaemia due to loss of blood because of the action of the parasites, a fact which completely changed the understanding of the pathology of the disorder.[45] As Wucherer stated, poor diet, alcohol, and unhygienic conditions could not account for the disorder as satisfactorily as the presence of parasites which, he speculated, were carried in water.[46] What had to be established were the conditions in which the parasite thrived and how these were related to climate. These were questions which Wucherer and his colleagues subsequently investigated. Significantly, Wucherer did not entirely discard factors such as poor diet and lack of hygiene, holding that they weakened the body and so predisposed it to the illness.

The disorder which Wucherer found has been identified as hookworm disease. The hookworm, anckylostoma, was first found by Angelo Dubini in Milan in 1838 but it was not until 1853 that Theodor Bilharz and Wilhem Griesinger, using Egyptian data, pointed to causal links between the worm and 'Egyptian chlorosis'.[47]

European doctors did not pick up on the insight for a long time because they were not particularly interested in the findings. It was, in fact, the building of the St Gotthard tunnel between the Italian and Swiss Alps, from 1880 to 1882, when scores of workers succumbed to an unknown 'chlorosis', that led European doctors to focus on hookworm.[48] Despite the lack of interest in mainstream European medicine, a number of European colonial physicians did maintain an interest in the disorder, as did Wucherer and his colleagues, and recognized it as a major health hazard in the regions where they worked. This group of widely dispersed doctors corresponded with each other, exchanged specimens, and generally kept alive investigations into the hookworm disorder for many years. By the time the mysterious 'chlorosis' which hit the St Gotthard tunnel workers had been diagnosed as hookworm disease a bank of information on hookworm-related disorders had been accumulated, part of which was contributed by the Brazilians.

If Wucherer, while advancing the shift over to the germ theory was reluctant to relinquish the environmental, in the writings of his disciple and young Tropicalista, Manoel Victorino Pereira, we see a blatantly eclectic bundling of disease aetiologies in order to satisfy his own political agenda for social reform. Of all the Tropicalistas Victorino Pereira was the most politically engaged and the most active campaigner against slavery, an institution he despised as a measure of Brazil's backwardness.[49] In reviewing Wucherer's work on 'hypoemia tropical', Victorino Pereira extolled the former's original contribution of highlighting the parasitical nature of the disorder. But he did not shed older notions of its aetiology. He wrote that environmental factors determined the reproduction of the worm in the host and of a particular individual becoming that host. After blaming environmental factors for the presence of the worm, if not for the cause of the illness, Victorino Pereira moved on to a scathing attack on the institution of slavery. After enumerating a list of abysmal conditions which were likely to promote the spread of the worm, he stated:

> The best preventive measure that I know of ... is to return to those miserable captives the liberty of which they were robbed, and to hand over the prodigious fertility of our lands and the incalculable wealth of our mines to the robust arms of free labour.... 'Hypoemia' [hookworm] is a disease of the poor, of the slaves, of the wretched.[50]

Victorino Pereira illustrates well the Tropicalistas' attempt to retain the environment as a moulding influence upon the health of the people. Certain environments or bad institutions operating within the tropics, tolerated by a lax and ignorant government, were conducive to the sickliness of the population. This approach placed the Tropicalistas squarely within the abolitionist camp on the question of slavery.[51] To the abolitionists' argument that slavery was a sign of backwardness and an obstacle to higher progress, the Tropicalistas added that slavery was an obstacle to the achievement of a healthier population so necessary to the advance of civilization, for slavery provided a milieu in which all the dangers of tropical climate were exacerbated rather than attenuated.

The Tropicalistas were by no means the only physicians in Brazil who took a critical stand on slavery and the government that endorsed it. What was new about the Tropicalistas was that, together with an older approach to disease and medicine, they juggled with a new and 'scientific' model which was shifting the focus of their scrutiny from the environment to the individual and specific disorders. It was the new aspect of their work which made them internationally known and which, in turn, gave them a more forceful identity as a medical movement to be taken seriously back home. But in their critique of domestic problems the Tropicalistas remained close to social medicine viewing disease and social conditions as inextricably interwoven, and calling upon the government to be more active in the removal of tropical miasmatic conditions, such as those identified with slavery. In the writings of the Tropicalistas, therefore, there was a constant tension between the doctors as part of an older tradition of medicine focusing on populations and conditions, and the doctors as participants in the ongoing shift towards specificity focusing upon specific exotic entities producing specific disorders in the individual.[52] There was also a tension between their wanting to find diseases distinctive to the tropics and their wish to say that there were no specific diseases in the tropics only universal disorders exacerbated by the climate. But for all their contradictions and shifts, there was a thematic unity in their writings which was the concern to understand how best to control and manipulate the disorders common in their tropical nation.

That Wucherer's work on hookworm signalled a marked departure from traditional Brazilian medicine, is seen in the degree of controversy his work generated. The leading expert on the disorder at the time was the Rio de Janeiro court physician, Cruz Jobim, who held closely to the notion of tropical miasma and topography as the cause of 'hypoemia tropical'. Such was the prestige of Dr Cruz Jobim that in 1867 the Imperial Academy of Medicine in Rio de Janeiro voted to reject Wucherer's hypothesis on rather unclear grounds. The confrontation between Cruz Jobim and Wucherer was a confrontation between an older theory of disease and a newly evolving one, as well as between a prestigious court physician and an unknown provincial one. But it was also a confrontation between two doctors in Brazil linked to different networks of European doctors. And herein lies another aspect of the novelty of the Tropicalistas.

Wucherer recognized hookworm because he was familiar with the work of Wilhelm Griesinger who had been one of his instructors at the University of Tubingen.[53] In Brazil Wucherer maintained his contacts with Griesinger with whom he regularly corresponded and exchanged specimens. Wucherer, like other Tropicalistas, also kept in touch with the German and English parasitologists, Rudolph Leuckhart and Spencer T. Cobbold, and with Le Roy Mericourt, a French naval doctor interested in the disorders of the tropical regions, as well as a number of other physicians around the world interested in the disorders of warm climates.[54] Indeed, it can be argued that the Tropicalistas were part of an informal network of geographically isolated doctor-scientists working in warm climates, and often focusing on parasites, who corresponded with each other, exchanged specimens, kept informed of one another's work through the medical journals, and who also, as Worboys has suggested, met up occasionally on their trips to European capitals and who were able to communicate because of their lack of specialization.[55] As is clear from the articles they chose to reproduce in their journal, the Tropicalistas were far more interested in the findings of a then relatively unknown Joseph Bancroft or Patrick Manson than in the leading exponents of European medicine. They found the former, working in warm climates, more relevant to their own situation. Thus, even while Europeans continued to be crucially important, the Tropicalistas chose to privilege some aspects of European medicine over others according to what they deemed most relevant to the requirements of their country. This was one of the main differences between an earlier generation of Brazilian doctors, such as Cruz Jobim, who preferred to replicate European medicine and European institutions as closely as possible in Brazil as a sign of the latter's advancement, and a later generation of doctors who saw themselves as part of an endeavour to use European methods and theories to promote original research. Like Europeans, this generation believed in science, but they looked to science produced in the tropics, *about* the tropics to help them confront what they saw as the distinctive problems of health and civilization in the 'torrid zone'.

Although individual members of the Tropicalistas continued to be prominent in their field until the end of the century, the Tropicalistas were ceasing to be a clearly defined group from the mid-1880s for several reasons. By then the Tropicalistas had gained the acceptance they sought moving from being obscure clinicians in a tropical backwater to becoming the founders of a prestigious journal cited in the international medical press, and the promoters of a shift of interest within Brazil from European medical concerns to Brazilian ones. However, their acceptance into the medical establishment also spelled the end of their distinctiveness as a movement. The Tropicalistas were never able fully to institutionalize their early ideal of pure medicine and research in the tropics in order to make a sustained contribution to medical science and to train disciples to carry on their work. Moreover, in the 1880s the Tropicalistas were caught up in the political struggles of a decade which saw the abolition of slavery in Brazil and the fall of the monarchy. Silva Lima's plaintive comment that his son-in-law, Victorino Pereira, should never have entered politics because in doing so he sacrificed his early promise of excellence in medical science, could just as well be read as a complaint about the Tropicalista movement itself.

A decade and a half later the attempt to institutionalize the scientific investigation of bacteriology in Rio de Janeiro under the leadership of Oswaldo Cruz had a most successful outcome.[56] There were many factors which enabled Cruz to set up a successful research institution, funded by the government. Crucial to his success was the relatively peaceful context of the Old Republic.[57] Perhaps even more important were the bacteriological advances of the 1880s and 1890s and the realization that governments could benefit economically by financing medical science. The model for successful medical research in this new era included official recognition and funding. At the time the Tropicalistas had set out on their journey of medical discovery, it had still been possible for doctor-scientists to hope for recognition, even fame, from their activities as freelance clinicians and researchers. The Tropicalistas failed to make the transition into an era of medicine which required far greater organization and funding than had been the case around mid-century.

Conclusion

In this paper I have attempted to make a contribution to the recent literature in the history of medicine by arguing that a number of our accepted ideas about the rise of tropical medicine should be re-examined to account not only for the European component but also for the ways in which dominant European ideas underwent adaptation in different regions around the world, through processes of selection, blending and fragmentation according to local requirements. I have argued that in the case of nineteenth-century Brazil, although there was a great deal of interplay between European and Brazilian medical ideas, we miss a true understanding of the relationship if we view Brazilian physicians as simply passively imitating dominant European ideas. In the second half of the nineteenth century, before the undisputed hegemony of the germ theory, and before the upsurge in interest in colonial/tropical medicine, there were physicians in Brazil attempting to articulate a distinctive medicine of warm climates. I have noted their tentativeness as they dealt with two dominant paradigms of disease, and I have argued that they went back and forth selectively, often, for us with hindsight, in a contradictory manner. But their criteria for selection was not contradictory. They were interested in promoting the idea of the malleability and adaptability of man in the tropics and, by extension, the possibility of progress in Brazil.

Notes

1. The literature is now large. Some important recent contributions include David Arnold (ed.), *Imperial Medicine and Indigenous Societies* (Manchester: Manchester University Press, 1988); R. MacLeod and M. Lewis (eds), *Disease, Medicine and Empire* (London: Routledge, 1988); John Farley, *Bilharzia: A History of Imperial Tropical Medicine* (Cambridge: Cambridge University Press, 1991); Maryinez Lyons, *The Colonial Disease: A Social History of Sleeping Sickness in Northern Zaire, 1900–1940* (Cambridge, New York: Cambridge University Press, 1992); Michael Worboys, 'British colonial medicine and tropical imperialism: A comparative perspective', in G. M. van Heteren *et al.* (eds) *Dutch Medicine in the Malay Archipelago, 1816–1942* (Amsterdam: Rodopi, 1989); *idem* 'The emergence and early development of parasitology', in K. S. Warren and J. Z. Bowers (eds), *Parasitology: A Global Perspective* (New York: Springer-Verlag, 1983), 1–18; Martin Shapiro, 'Medicine in the service of colonialism: medical care in Portuguese Africa, 1885–1974', Ph.D. Dissertation, University of California, Los Angeles, 1983. For a recent work on tropical medicine before Manson see, Mark Harrison, 'Tropical medicine in nineteenth-century India', *British Journal for the History of Science,* 22 (1992), 299–318; the papers given at the conference on 'Tropical Medicine before Manson: Warm Climates and Western Medicine, *c.*1500–1900', London, Wellcome Institute, 25–26 March, 1993; Michael Worboys, 'From "Diseases in the Tropics" to "Tropical Diseases"', paper at conference on 'Disease and Society in the Developing World: Exploring New Perspectives', College of Physicians, Philadelphia, 24–26 September, 1992.

2. The first permanent universities were set up in 1551 in Peru and Mexico.
3. I am not suggesting that there has been no work whatsoever on Latin America. Some important research has been carried out as can be seen, for example, in Stepan's study on the Oswaldo Cruz Institute in Brazil and its contributions to tropical medicine in the early decades of this century. A more recent example is Cueto's well-handled study of the eradication of yellow fever in northern Peru in which he discusses the complex problem of Western medicine and technology in relation to local traditions and political resistance. What is common to the existing body of research into the history of tropical medicine in Latin America is that it deals with tropical medicine *after* the rise of the germ theory of disease, and *after* the great expansion of the imperial powers. Indeed, the episodes I have just referred to are the result of the internationalization of tropical medicine and North American philanthropy. In his campaign to stem the threat of bubonic plague and to eradicate yellow fever in Rio de Janeiro, for example, Oswaldo Cruz used as his model the US army's methods of sanitizing Havana. In Peru, the Rockefeller Foundation shaped the most crucial aspects of the campaign against yellow fever. Marcos Cueto, 'Sanitation from above: Yellow fever and foreign Intervention in Peru, 1919–1922', *Hispanic American Historical Review,* 72, (1992), 1–22; Nancy Leys Stepan, *Beginnings of Brazilian Science: Oswaldo Cruz, Medical Research and Policy, 1890–1920* (New York: Science History Publications, 1976). Recent works in the history of medicine and public health in Latin America include, Nancy Leys Stepan, *'The Hour of Eugenics': Race, Gender and Nation in Latin America* (Ithaca & London: Cornell University Press, 1991); *idem,* 'Initiation and survival of medical research in a developing country: The Oswaldo Cruz Institute of Brazil, 1900–1920', *Journal of the History of Medicine and Allied Sciences,* 30 (1975), 303–25; *idem,* 'The interplay between socio-economic factors and medical science: Yellow fever research, Cuba, and the United States', *Social Studies of Science,* 8 (1978), 397–423; Marcos Cueto, 'Excellence in the Periphery: Scientific Activities and Biomedical Sciences in Peru', Ph.D. Dissertation, Columbia University, 1988; 'The Rockefeller Foundation's medical policy and scientific research in Latin America: The case of physiology', *Social Studies of Science,* 20 (1990), 229–54; 'Visions of science and development: The Rockefeller Foundation's Latin American Surveys of the 1920s' in Moros Cueto (ed.), *Missionaries of Sèrence: The Rockefeller Foundation and Latin America* (Bloomington: Indiana University Press, 1994), 1–22. Luiz Antonio de Castro-Santos, 'Power, ideology, and public health in Brazil, 1889–1930', Ph.D. Dissertation, Harvard University, 1987; Armando Solorzano, 'The Rockefeller Foundation in Mexico: Nationalism, public health, and yellow fever (1911–1924)', Ph.D. Dissertation, University of Wisconsin-Madison, 1990; Robin L.

Anderson, 'Public health and public healthiness, Sao Paulo, Brazil, 1876–1893', *Journal of the History of Medicine,* 41 (1986), 293–307; Sam C. Adamo, 'The broken promise: Race, health, justice in Rio de Janeiro, 1890–1940', Ph.D. Dissertation, University of New Mexico, 1983; Ilana Lowy, 'Yellow fever in Rio de Janeiro and the Pasteur Institute Mission (1901–1905): The transfer of science to the periphery', *Medical History,* 34 (1990), 144–63; Donald Cooper, 'Brazil's long fight against epidemic disease, 1849–1907, with special emphasis on yellow fever', *Bulletin of the New York Academy of Medicine* 91, (1975), 672–96; 'The new "black death": Cholera in Brazil, 1855–56', *Social Science History,* 10 (1986) 467–88; Ron Mineo, 'Misery and death in the Pearl of the Pacific: Health care in Guayaquil, Ecuador, 1870–1925', *Hispanic American Historical Review,* 70, (1990), 609–37; Teresa Meade and Mark Walker (eds), *Science, Medicine, and Cultural Imperialism* (New York: St Martin's Press, 1991); Susanne Austin Alchon, *Native Society and Disease in Colonial Ecuador* (Cambridge & New York: Cambridge University Press, 1991); Kenneth F. Kiple, 'Cholera and Race in the Caribbean' *Journal of Latin American Studies,* 17 (1985), 157–77; James D. Goodyear, 'Agents of empire: Portuguese doctors in colonial Brazil and the idea of tropical disease', Ph.D. Dissertation, Johns Hopkins University, 1982; Noble David Cook and W. George Lovell (eds), *'Secret Judgements of God': Old World Disease in Colonial Spanish America* (Norman & London: University of Oklahoma Press, 1992); R. dos Santos, Piso e a *Medicina Indigena* (Pernambuco, 1980).

4. David Arnold, 'Europe's medicine overseas, 1500–1900', paper given at the conference on 'Tropical Medicine before Manson: Warm Climates and Western Medicine, *c.*1500–1900' London, Wellcome Institute, 25–26 March, 1993, 4.
5. For example, Fernando de Azevedo, *Brazilian Culture: An Introduction to the Study of Culture in Brazil,* trans. William Rex Crawford (New York: The Macmillan Company, 1950), 179–82, 423; Antonio Caldas Coni, *A Escola Tropicalista Bahiana* (Bahia, Brazil: Livraria Progresso, 1952).
6. Arnold, *op. cit.* (note 4), 4.
7. Benedict Anderson, *Imagined Communities: Reflections on the Origin and Spread of Nationalism* (London & New York: Verso, 1983), 15, 50–65.
8. On this question of tropical diseases as distinct from European ones, the doctors were often contradictory. Sometimes they affirmed that the disorders of hot climates were distinctive but there are also times when they seem to be saying the opposite. For example, the Tropicalistas were adamant that categorizing tuberculosis as a disease of temperate regions was erroneous and that it was very common in Brazil. In the 1880s they were quick to note that hookworm, found in the St Gotthard tunnel workers in Switzerland, had usually been

seen as a disease of the tropics.

9. On the War of the Triple Alliance against Paraguay, see E. Bradford Burns, *A History of Brazil* (New York: Columbia University Press, 1980), 231–6.
10. On the empire years in Brazil, see Emilia Viotti da Costa, *The Brazilian Empire: Myths and Histories* (Chicago & London: The University of Chicago Press, 1985).
11. One of the ways in which the Tropicalistas saw themselves as breaking with the tradition of Brazilian medicine was that they argued that a doctor's influence should arise from his scientific expertise and not from his preeminence in the patronage network or political arena. They were not entirely successful in making this shift.
12. For medical education under the Brazilian Empire see Primitivo Moacyr, *A Instrucçao e o Imperio (Subsidios para a História da Educaçao no Imperio) 1854–1889* 3 vols, (São Paulo: 1938); Lycurgo Santos Filho, *História da Medicina no Brasil* 2 vols, (Sao Paulo: Editora Brasiliense, 1947); Gilberto Freyre, *Order and Progress: Brazil from Monarch to Republic,* trans. Rod W. Horton (Berkeley: University of California Press, 1986), 103–65. There were two medical schools in Brazil during the Empire set up in 1808 in Salvador, Bahia and Rio de Janeiro.
13. Erwin H. Ackerknecht, *A Short History of Medicine,* (New York: The Ronald Press Co., 1955), 157.
14. For example, 'Patologia interna sobre a molestia vulgarmente denominada opilação ou cansanço', *Gazeta Médica da Bahia,* 1 (1866), 27–9, 39–41, 52–4, 63–4. See following note for other titles.
15. Otto Wucherer, 'Nota Preliminar, sobre Vermes de uma Especie ainda nao Descripta, Encontrados na Urina de Doentes de Hematuria Intertropical no Brasil', *ibid.,* 3 (1868), 97–9 and 'Sobre a hematuria no Brasil', *ibid.,* 4, (1869), 39–40, 49–50, 61–2, 73–4, 85–6.
16. For example, the French doctor Sigaud who wrote one of the most important books in the nineteenth century about the disorders of Brazil, *Du climat et des maladies de Bresil; ou statistique medicale de cet empire* (Paris: Fortin, Masson, 1844); T. J. H. Langaard who wrote, *Diccionario de Medicina* (1865); Aristides Garnier, a Frenchman who lived in Rio de Janeiro and directed the journal of the Brazilian Academy of Medicine, *Annais Brasilienses de Medicina;* the Englishman, Jonathon Abbot who taught and worked in Bahia and founded a small natural history museum in the Bahian Medical School.
17. For changes in clinical medicine in this period see, Kenneth D. Keele, 'Clinical Medicine in the 1860s', in F. N. L. Poynter, (ed.), *Medicine and Science in the 1860s* (London: Wellcome Institute for the History of Medicine, 1968), 1–11.
18. On the Santa Casa, see A. J. R. Russell-Wood, *Fidalgos and Philanthropists: The Santa Casa de Misericordia of Bahia, 1550–1755* (Berkeley & Los Angeles: University of California Press, 1968);

Carlos Ott, *A Santa Casa de Misericordia da Cidade do Salvador* (Rio de Janeiro: 1960); Julyan G. Peard, 'The Tropicalista School of Medicine of Bahia, Brazil, 1860–1889', Ph.D. Dissertation, University of Columbia 1990, 48–53.

19. The Tropicalistas were very interested in Brazilian pharmacopoeia. This is a subject which deserves further investigation. Thomas Glick has argued that European visitors to America, especially Humboldt, contributed to the idea that Latin Americans might develop their own scientific enterprise, some advocating the idea of developing an American pharmacopoeia. This hope was checked by the wars of independence when many doctors and naturalists in Latin America were killed. Even in Brazil, where independence came relatively peacefully, the problems of nationhood took up much of the energies of the few scientific men and the perception of Latin American instability probably stopped European naturalists from going to that continent. Although the Tropicalistas wrote a number of articles on the subject of local remedies, and called for more research on the subject, it never became a central focus for them. For some of their writings, see Peard, *op. cit.* (note 18), 100, note 116. On science and independence see Thomas F. Glick, 'Science and independence in Latin America (with special reference to New Granada)', *Hispanic American Historical Review,* 71, (1991), 307–34.
20. Peard, *op. cit.* (note 18), 70–1.
21. *Gazeta Médica da Bahia,* 6 (1872).
22. As argued, for example, by Louis Agassiz and Arthur Gobineau, two nineteenth-century visitors to Brazil. See Thomas E. Skidmore, *Black into White: Race, Nationality, and Brazilian Thought* (New York: Oxford University Press, 1974).
23. 'Contribução para a historia de uma molestia que reina na Bahia sob a forma epidemica e caracterizada por paralisia, edema e fraqueza geral', *Gazeta Médica da Bahia,* 1 (1866) 110–13, 125–8, 138–9, 158–60, 183–5, 196–8, 219–20, 232–5, 243–5, 268–70; (1867), 2–6, 28–30, 49–55, 65–8, 99–104; (1868), 55–6, 85–7, 109–11. In 1872 the articles were published in book form with the title, *Ensaio sobre o Beriberi no Brasil* (Salvador: 1872).
24. His subsequent reading was mainly on the work of British doctors in India such as C. Morehead, *Clinical Researches on Disease in India* Vol. II, (London: Longman, 1856). He also read the work of Aitken and, in French publications, writings by Monneret de la Berge and Fonssagrives.
25. The numbers he gave for his 'epidemic' were very small. On the definition of epidemic in the nineteenth century see Lyons *op. cit.* (note 1), who has noted that at the time epidemic meant not so much disorders transmitted from sick to healthy but which simultaneously affected people because of atmospheric conditions.
26. On the concept of miasma, see Charles-Edward Amory Winslow, *The*

Conquest of Epidemic Disease: A Chapter in the History of Ideas (Madison: University of Wisconsin Press, 1980); Dennis G. Carlson, *African Fever: A Study of British Science, Technology and Politics in West Africa, 1787–1864* (Canton, Ma.: Science History Publications, 1984); Owsei Temkin, 'A historical analysis of the concept of infection', in *idem, The Double Face of Janus* (Baltimore & London: The Johns Hopkins University Press, 1977); Nancy Tomes, 'The private side of health: Sanitary science, domestic hygiene, and the germ theory, 1870–1900', *Bulletin of the History of Medicine,* 64 (1990), 503–39.

27. Silva Lima, 'Contribuçăo', *Gazeta Médica da Bahia* (1867), 101.
28. *Ibid.,* 102–3. A most plausible observation as only upper-class Brazilians would have been able to afford the more polished, and thus less nutritious, white rice at this time.
29. Silva Lima, 'Noticias acerca do Kakke, ou beriberi das Indias orientais', *Gazeta Médica da Bahia,* 12 (1888), 387; for an interesting treatment of the theoretical compatibility between the germ theory and miasma see Tomes, *op. cit.* (note 26), 514–15, 528–30.
30. Antonio Pacifico Pereira, 'Estudio sobre a etiologia e naturaleza do beriberi', *Gazeta Médica da Bahia,* 12 (1881), 308–17, 453–62, 485–98, 533–43; 13 (1882), 1–12, 49–66, 97–106, 145–53, 193–200, 308–17, 409–19, 496–502.
31. *Ibid.,* 12 (1881), 533–4.
32. *Ibid.,* 13 (1881), 9–10.
33. *Ibid.,* 12 (1881): 535–6.
34. Antonio Pacifico Pereira, 'Hygiene das escolas', *Gazeta Médica da Bahia,* 10 (1878), 252, emphasis added. The importance of ventilation was a very old theme in Western medicine and in tropical disease: see John J. Keevil, Christopher Lloyd and Jack L. Coulter (eds), *Medicine and the Navy, 1200–1900,* Vol. IV (Edinburgh and London: E & S Livingstone, 1963), 81–90.
35. *Gazeta Médica da Bahia,* 10 (1878), 193–201, 241–52, 289–95, 337–47, 433–49; Peard, *op. cit.* (note 18), 344–63.
36. *Gazeta Médica da Bahia,* 10 (1878), 252. As the implications of Pasteur's theory began to be understood, many doctors in Brazil and elsewhere claimed to have found the bacteriological causes of some of the most common and puzzling diseases of the time. For Brazil see Lowy, *op. cit.* (note 3),
37. It is interesting to note that when sections of Pereira's article were reproduced in the foreign press it was his findings on micro-organisms that were most commented upon. See 'Pereira on the blood in beriberi', *London Medical Record,* 10 (1882), 464–5; *St. Louis Medical & Surgical Journal,* 42 (1882), 25–38, 263–6, 365–8, 590–3.
38. See the exchange between Pacifico Pereira and J. B. de Lacerda, 'Investigaçóes sobre o Beriberi', *Gazeta Médica da Bahia* 15 (1883), 159–70 and 'O Micro-Organismo do Beriberi', *ibid.,* 312.

39. Pereira, *op. cit.* (note 38), 159–70.
40. He was not alone in his balancing act. As Ackerknecht has noted, there existed a large number of physicians, whom he called 'contingent contagionists', who, in theory, allowed that epidemics might be caused by contagion (through 'fomites' and later through bacteria) but who in their practical considerations, followed the miasmatists in advocating cleaning up the environment in order to destroy the miasmatic emanations which caused disease. E.H. Ackerknecht, 'Anticontagionism between 1821 and 1867', *Bulletin of the History of Medicine,* 22 (1948), 562–93.
41. A. Pacheco Mendes, 'Contribução ao estudo do beriberi', *Gazeta Médica da Bahia,* 16 (1884), 129–35, 157–60, 208–13, 260–4.
42. Eric Cassell has argued that the tension between these two views is present even today, 'Ideas in conflict: The rise and fall (and rise and fall) of new views of disease', *Daedalus,* 115, (1986), 21–22; on the differentiation between the 'old' tropical medicine and the 'new' in Brazil, see Lowy, *op. cit.* (note 3), 161–3.
43. Also known in Brazil as 'opilaç̄ao' and 'cansanço'. The disorder was known in various parts of the world as: 'cachexia africana', 'tropical chlorosis', 'mal d'estomac', 'mal de coeur': Erwin H. Ackerknecht, *History and Geography of the Most Important Diseases* (London & New York: Harper Publishing Co., 1965), 130.
44. Otto Wucherer, 'Patologia interna sobre a molestia vulgarmente denominada opilaçao ou cansanco', *Gazeta Médica da Bahia,* 1 (1866), 27–9, 39–41, 52–4, 63–4.
45. There is a discrepancy in the historical and medical literature as to who were the main victims of the disorder. In Brazil the disease was always associated with slaves and field workers whereas in North America and the Caribbean, what is believed to have been hookworm, was viewed as successfully resisted by Blacks and contracted more easily by Whites. The Tropicalistas held that most of the victims of the disease were the poorest elements of the society.
46. *Gazeta Médica da Bahia,* 1 (1866), 27.
47. H.Harold Scott, *A History of Tropical Medicine,* Vol. II, (Baltimore: Williams & Wilkins Company, 1930), 841.
48. Ackerknecht, *op. cit.* (note 43), 131–2. Wucherer's work on hookworm was first published in Europe in Germany by Griesinger who communicated the results of Wucherer's work to *Archiv für Heilkunde* (1866), 387.
49. Manoel Victorino Pereira became Vice-President of the Republic in the 1890s shortly after the fall of the Brazilian Empire. He was also one of the leaders of the Liberal party in Bahia and an active abolitionist.
50. Manoel Victorino Pereira, 'Anckylostoma duodenale, Chlorose de Egypto – Hypoemia Tropical', *Gazeta Médica da Bahia,* 9 (1876), 78, 81.

51. For the abolition of Brazilian slavery, see Rebecca J. Scott *et al.*, *The Abolition of Slavery and the Aftermath of Emancipation in Brazil* (Durham & London: Duke University Press, 1988).
52. Elizabeth Fee deals with the practical implications in the different styles in the ways of understanding and studying diseases in, 'Sin versus science: Venereal disease in twentieth century Baltimore', in Elizabeth Fee and Daniel Fox (eds), *AIDS: The Burdens of History* (Berkeley: University of California Press, 1988), 121–46.
53. Caldas Coni, *Escola Tropicalista,* 45
54. T. Spencer Cobbold, *Parasites: A Treatise on the Entozoa of Man and Animals* (London: J. & A. Churchill, 1879), 213–15.
55. Worboys, 'Emergence and early development of parasitology', (note 1), 5.
56. Stepan, *op. cit.* (note 3), 84–101.
57. Despite the threats to its stability that the Old Republic faced from millenarian movements, urban rebellions and struggles between regional oligarchies, it was still a government consolidating its power with a clearly defined approach to the role that scientists should play in the nation. This contrasted with the final decades of the Empire when the government was losing its legitimacy and was unclear about the role that science and research should play in the nation.

7

A Question of Locality: The Identity of Cholera in British India, 1860–1890

Mark Harrison

The rapid and pervasive dissemination of cholera during the nineteenth century appears to provide a graphic illustration of what Emmanuel Le Roy Ladurie has termed 'the unification of the globe by disease'.[1] The spread of cholera from its 'home' in Lower Bengal – along the caravan routes of Central Asia, around the rim of the Indian Ocean, and to the Middle East with Muslim pilgrims to Mecca – brought a heightened awareness of the extent to which the fate of nations was interconnected.[2] Cholera met with an unprecedented international response: from 1851 through to the end of the century, no less than ten International Sanitary Conferences were staged with the object of agreeing quarantine and other measures to stem the spread of the disease.[3] But, despite the fact that cholera had appeared in epidemic form in most major trading countries or their colonies by the end of the nineteenth century, it was still perceived as an alien and, often, a specifically Indian disease.[4]

The persistent image of cholera as an 'Asiatic' disease, of course, reflected the fact that India was its place of origin. Yet, as I hope to demonstrate, this continuing association also owed something to a distinctive British–Indian medical tradition,[5] which claimed cholera as its own, as well as to the political implications of admitting that cholera was a truly international disease. Against mounting opposition from its own medical officers, and in the face of scorn and ridicule abroad, the Government of India maintained the traditional British–Indian view that the subcontinent was epidemiologically unique: that cholera behaved differently in India compared with the other countries in which it had appeared.[6] Cholera, it claimed, was an Indian disease and foreign experts had no business meddling in British India's affairs.

Cholera, and the question of its mode of spread, impinged on some of the most important and problematic areas of colonial administration.[7] The notion that cholera was, in some sense, a 'contagious' disease – whether transmitted directly from person to person, or indirectly in contaminated food and water – was the basis for most international action against the disease. The quarantines and other measures imposed against Indian shipping in Europe and the Suez Canal had a damaging effect on India's trade. Being aimed primarily at the Hadj – the annual pilgrimage of Muslims to Mecca and Medina – these measures also created profound difficulties for the Government of India, which had been seeking the cooperation of Indian Muslim élites.[8]

But the question of cholera dissemination had other important political ramifications. Delegates to International Sanitary Conferences demanded stricter measures to control the spread of cholera *within* India, including the regulation of internal pilgrimages. Cholera was also at the heart of debates about the administration of India and, in particular, the question of the government's responsibility for public health. The Government of India became synonymous with sanitary neglect and the target of reformers both in Britain and in India. These reformers attacked the very foundation of the government's position on cholera, with an assault on its primarily localist and atmospheric notions of causation and transmission. Stressing the special danger of water, and the need for government to finance large water-purification schemes, their demands ran contrary both to official doctrine and moves to decentralize and reduce government expenditure.

Before discussing in more detail the political implications of cholera's geographical identity, it is worth considering the 'identity' of disease in its broadest sense. Scholars such as François Delaporte and Michael Worboys have recently stressed the importance of understanding disease in terms of cultural practices rather than as a simple biological entity.[9] Viewed in this way, the identity of a disease is often indistinguishable from measures taken to control it. Charles Rosenberg also views disease as being constructed in a complex nexus 'between biological event, and its perception by patient and practitioner' as well as the 'collective effort to make cognitive and policy sense out of these perception'.[10] More recently, Andrew Cunningham has suggested that a disease is defined by the answers people (patients, practitioners, etc.) give to questions which are asked about it.[11] These definitions represent an important shift away from a narrowly medical and biologically reductionist view of disease as an unchanging entity. They all stress, to varying extents, the historical contingency of our understanding of disease. But the question remains: how and in what ways do the views of historical actors shape the construction of disease? Following the work of Bruno Latour,[12] there has been a tendency, evident in the work of Cunningham for example, merely to identify the various actors involved in defining a disease, without considering the economic, political and professional interests which may have moulded their outlook. Indeed, Latour considers such an enterprise illegitimate, since he claims that 'interests' are indistinguishable from the claims which actors make.

To take the claims of actors at face value would obviously be naive but to conceive of 'interests' in this way is to misunderstand what is usually meant by the term in the sociology and history of science and medicine. Interests have traditionally been understood not as the self-proclaimed goals of actors but the socio-political factors which have a bearing upon an individual's world view. Latour's conception of the construction of medical knowledge is too detached to bear historical fruit.[13]

In this essay I have attempted to identify the interests of various constituencies in the Indian cholera debate in a way that avoids the rigid dichotomies ('contagionist/anticontagionist', 'liberal/conservative') which characterized early attempts to locate cholera theory and practices within a political and economic framework.[14] The inadequacies of such rigid distinctions have been pointed out elsewhere.[15] Rather, following Delaporte, I have adopted a more flexible view which attempts to understand why various interests – professional, political and economic – coalesce around a particular view of disease at a given point in time.

'The Special Geography of Hindoostan'

To enter the realm of medical theory in India in the 1860s and 1870s is to enter the abstract world of Dr James Lumsdaine Bryden (1833–80). Bryden, an MD of Edinburgh University, became the first person to occupy the post of Statistical Officer to the Government of India's newly formed Sanitary Department.[16] Having gained first-hand experience of cholera as a civil surgeon in Bengal, where the disease was endemic, Bryden had been well placed to observe its seasonal fluctuations and its seemingly law-like behaviour under Indian conditions.

Soon after being appointed Statistical Officer, Bryden was commissioned by the government to investigate the phenomenon of *epidemic* cholera. His main tasks were to establish the geographical limits of the disease, the duration of epidemics, the influence of meteorological conditions and, most importantly, its mode of propagation and spread. Bryden's enterprise was such that he and commentators in the medical press came to refer to it as a 'natural history' of cholera:[17] a form of enquiry which had its roots in eighteenth-century natural philosophy, with its emphasis on adaptation to the environment, and the need to understand natural phenomena from a historical perspective.[18]

Newtonian physics had given new life to the notion that nature was a coherent and interconnected whole and that most, perhaps all, physical phenomena were governed by natural laws.[19] Bryden believed that the essential nature of these laws was beyond human understanding but that they were capable of being measured and manipulated for the benefit of humanity.[20] The task of the 'natural historian' was to gather as much data as possible relating to the object of the study and its physical surroundings. From these data he would attempt to deduce the law governing the phenomena under observation. It was an attempt to impose order on the natural world – in Bryden's case, on an alien and seemingly hostile environment. In this respect, Bryden's statistical reports formed part of a much wider endeavour. Together with the geological, botanical, zoological and meteorological surveys of India, medical men aimed to understand the Indian environment and render it habitable and bountiful for Europeans.[21]

The Enlightenment tradition filtered down to Bryden through three sources: his medical training at Edinburgh, from existing work on tropical hygiene and medical topography in India, and the legacy of William Farr, Compiler of Abstracts at the Registrar-General's office in London. Farr, who was appointed in 1839, had made a number of prophetic deductions about the course of epidemics from epidemiological data.[22] His work almost certainly provided the model for Bryden in India. He adopted Farr's Liebigian nosology and his statistical methods, and shared his conviction that all physical phenomena were essentially law-abiding and capable of being predicted.[23] For Bryden and Farr statistics were the 'Sibylline books of modern times ... an unerring guide to the future'.[24]

But Bryden differed from Farr in one crucial respect. By 1866 Farr's observations had led him to believe that cholera was spread in contaminated drinking water, but, until his death, Bryden remained convinced that cholera was an air- and not a waterborne disease.[25] Bryden believed that there were two processes at work in the generation of epidemic cholera. The first was that the pathogenic organism – which he likened to a seed – underwent a cycle of reproduction and decay which was quickened or retarded by certain environmental conditions. The second was the phenomenon of epidemic spread itself, in which cholera seeds were transported beyond the endemic area by monsoonal air currents. With this in mind, Bryden produced a topography of cholera, representing graphically the limits of epidemic influence.

Meteorological conditions were the key determinants of these epidemic zones, affecting both the vitality and the mobility of the cholera seed. He maintained that the 'vehicle is in all cases, and whenever epidemic advance is in progress, a humid atmosphere'. The prevailing wind was the agency which directed the course of an epidemic and determined its limitation in geographical distribution.[26] The perennial coincidence of certain meteorological phenomena combined with the fact that India was the only country in which the disease was endemic gave rise to the belief that India was epidemiologically unique. 'It is the special geography of Hindoostan', insisted Bryden, 'the regularity with which the seasons come forward year after year, and the normality of the limit of the meteorological agencies in every year that causes its surface to became mapped into normal areas.'[27]

Bryden's views on cholera causation were shared by other senior officers of the Indian Medical Service (IMS). The Sanitary Commissioner with the Government of India from 1866 to 1884, James McNabb Cuningham (1829–1905), was another Edinburgh graduate and personally well-disposed to Bryden and his attempt to adduce a general law of cholera dissemination. Like Bryden, Cuningham apparently 'relied more on statistics than on research' and was 'apt to throw cold water on strivings towards the truth by local inquiry and clinical and pathological investigation'.[28] In Cuningham's hands, Bryden's localist/atmospheric theory of cholera epidemics became a powerful tool against advocates of quarantine and those who pressed government to intervene more directly in public health.

'Fallacious Statistics and Wild Schemes'

The government's most persistent critic was Annesley Charles DeRenzy (1828–1914), Sanitary Commissioner of the Punjab. A partisan of Snow's waterborne theory, DeRenzy mounted a concerted attack on Bryden's hypothesis and on government for its inaction in the sphere of public health.[29] DeRenzy drew his inspiration and his model of sanitary reform from Britain, and cited metropolitan authorities in his attacks upon the colonial medical establishment. 'I had two special reasons for examining Dr Bryden's theory', he explained in a letter defending one of his annual reports,

> first it is calculated to severely retard sanitary progress ... second, it has been the basis of the action of the Government of India against cholera.... To substantiate the first reason, I have only to refer to almost every review of Dr Bryden's book. It will suffice to quote here the opinion of one whose authority is universally admitted, Dr Parkes. He says – 'Dr Bryden's views strike at the heart of the usual preventive measures'.[30]

Parkes, like most medical men in Britain, had come to believe in the efficacy of more specific measures against cholera. He recommended chemical examination of drinking water and its purification by the addition of substances like alum and filtration through sand and charcoal.[31] Bryden saw no need for special attention regarding the water supply. He thought it detracted from the main object of sanitation – the removal of the filth in which the cholera seed was thought to propagate. The only additional measure deemed useful against cholera by Bryden was the improvement of barracks and European dwellings to guard against aerial incursions by the disease.

DeRenzy recognized the need for adequate accommodation for troops in India but protested strongly against other items of sanitary expenditure, especially about the large sums of money expended on the administration of the Contagious Diseases Act. He believed that the money would be better spent on improvements to the water supply in cantonments and in grants-in-aid to municipal commissions.[32] Prior to DeRenzy's crusade, very few IMS officers singled out the water supply as the 'favoured' medium of cholera and DeRenzy readily acknowledged that Bryden's theory held sway among medical men in India.[33]

DeRenzy and the Government of India first crossed swords in 1870, over the former's unfavourable review of Bryden's treatise on cholera. 'Dr DeRenzy', protested the government's Sanitary Commissioner,

> does but scant justice to Dr Bryden's remarkable work; and it appears to me that if such a proceeding be generally followed, it will lead to very inconvenient results. I would therefore strongly recommend that the Sanitary Commissioners refrain from criticizing the views held by other officers of the same Department.[34]

But DeRenzy did not refrain from criticizing Bryden and, in 1872, the Government of India made a formal protest to DeRenzy's superiors. DeRenzy was 'instructed to adhere strictly to the orders of the Government of India in the presentation of future reports'.[35]

Indeed, DeRenzy appears to have courted unpopularity on a grand scale. As well as the Government of India, he had incurred the wrath of his local newspaper, the *Indian Public Opinion and Punjab Times,* which accused him of neglecting his duty during a cholera epidemic in the province, during which he been in the hills collecting statistics for his cholera research. The newspaper had referred to 'his fallacious statistics and wild schemes', and his 'love of the hills when his duty was in the plains'. A correspondent to the newspaper, Dr Taylor, also imputed that DeRenzy had lacked courage in departing from Amritsar during an outbreak of the disease. Outraged by these allegations, DeRenzy took the *Punjab Times* to court, suing the newspaper for Rs 1,000, but obtaining damages of only Rs 500; a verdict that suggested that the newspaper's claims had not been entirely without substance.[36] More significant is the nature of the claims themselves: DeRenzy seems to have been regarded as a zealot, or at least as some kind of crank, whose views on cholera were unrepresentative of British–Indian opinion.

But DeRenzy was not alone in his criticism of government, or in his support for Snow's waterborne theory. 'At no time', wrote the Secretary to the Bengal government, 'has controversy on the causation of the disease [cholera] run higher than at the present'.[37] Unfortunately for Cuningham, who was at that time defending his new department from critics within the general IMS, much of this dissent came from within its own ranks. The Sanitary Commissioner of the North-West Provinces, for example, took a stance on cholera which emphasized 'contagion' to a much greater extent than Cuningham and Bryden. 'The chief prevalence of the disease in a cluster of villages', he concluded, 'seems to point to contagion as one cause of the spread, whilst prevalence in isolated centres of population may point to local insanitary conditions as the cause of the outbreak'.[38] Dr Coates, Sanitary Commissioner for Bengal, was also of the opinion that 'to limit the cause of cholera to any one factor and its entrance into the system would be unwise'. Yet he was moving increasingly towards the position of DeRenzy and Snow. 'My conviction', he wrote in his annual report of 1878, 'has become stronger and stronger that there is a connection between impure water and the disease'.[39]

There were dissentient voices, too, outside of the Sanitary Department. 'Dr Bryden', wrote the editor of the *Indian Medical Gazette* in 1872,

> with a bold combination of the philosophy of Aristotle and Pythagoras has, in recent years, furnished us with a striking illustration of a reversion to a metaphysical stage of scientific thought.... He rejects the tedious system of elaborating principles and well observed instances. Principles thus obtained are secondary truths.[40]

He felt that Bryden's mode of inquiry, though nominally empirical, tended towards unnecessary and somewhat inflexible theorizing about the 'laws' which seemed to govern cholera. The *Gazette*'s editor concurred in DeRenzy's view that the existence of local factors in cholera causation was not inconsistent with the communicability of the disease, but expressed regret that he had detected some acerbity in his tone. 'When will doctors', he lamented, 'learn to differ amiably'.[41]

In Britain too, since the Army Sanitary Commission's unfavourable report of 1863, there was concern that the Government of India was not doing enough to protect British troops from disease.[42] Some, like Florence Nightingale, extended their critical gaze to 'reservoirs of disease' outside military cantonments. Like a growing number of Britons in India, she advocated a more interventionist sanitary programme financed partly by local taxation and partly by government. For Nightingale and others of her ilk, the cleansing of India was both a humanitarian duty and a military necessity.[43]

A Disease of Locality

These criticisms came at a time when the Government of India was attempting to distance itself from matters of public health. From 1870, under the administration of Lord Mayo (Governor-General from 1869 to 1872), the political climate was in no sense conducive to sanitary reform. Mayo had inherited a large budgetary deficit from the expansionist regime of Lord Lawrence (1863–9) which he sought to remedy by increasing taxation and reducing public expenditure.[44] A key part of Mayo's strategy, and one which received the full backing of the first Gladstone government, was his Resolution on Provincial Finance of 1870. Its aim was to give provincial governments an incentive to cut public spending by devolving upon them certain heads of income and expenditure previously controlled by the Indian government.[45] Provincial governments, in turn, were keen to see the burden of sanitary expenditure shouldered by the municipalities and, with this in mind, the elective principle was reintroduced in municipal commissions in some of the major towns.

The other issue which focused attention on cholera at this time was the controversy surrounding the epidemic of 1867 – the first major outbreak of the disease since the report of the Royal Commission on the Health of the Army in India in 1863. Originating in Hurdwar in the North-West Provinces, where thousands of pilgrims had gathered for the Kumbh Mela (a religious fair), the epidemic appeared to spread outwards along the routes of returning pilgrims, affecting towns and military cantonments. The direct threat posed to the health of European troops, and the demand by delegates to the Constantinople sanitary conference that the Indian government make sanitary provisions at places of pilgrimage within India, led the government to launch an inquiry into the causes of the 1867 epidemic.[46]

The two persons chosen to conduct the enquiry were Bryden and Dr John Murray (1809–98), Inspector-General of Hospitals for the North-West Provinces. Bryden's nomination was not surprising given his position as Statistical Officer to the Sanitary Department, but Murray was something of an unknown quantity, having hitherto displayed no special interest in cholera.[47] Much to the government's annoyance, the two investigators came to very different conclusions about how the disease was spread. Some sections of their joint report reveal the meteorological bias of Bryden, while others reflect the contingent-contagionist perspective of Dr Murray. 'It cannot be regarded as mere coincidence', wrote one of its authors (presumably Murray),

> that in thirty-five districts of Upper-India ... the epidemic should have gradually appeared in one place after another, immediately after the return of a body of pilgrims stricken by the disease.... Without a doubt, the germ of epidemic cholera appears to reside in the evacuations of a person suffering from the disease.[48]

Murray went on to recommend strict regulation of the water supply and restrictions on population movement as preventives against cholera. He envisaged a system whereby special camps supplied with pure water and hospital accommodation would be set up at regular intervals to and from religious gatherings, averting the need for pilgrims to enter cantonments or towns in search of accommodation or sustenance. Murray also believed that there was a role for conventional *cordons sanitaires* whenever 'unusual danger' threatened.[49]

Murray's recommendations, which were reiterated by the MacKenzie Committee commissioned by the Madras government, appear to have been rejected by the Indian government on grounds of cost.[50] However, public order considerations were almost certainly as important, since there is some evidence to show that even the basic sanitary measures introduced at the Kumbh Mela were not popular among pilgrims.

According to Drs Bryden and Murray:

> the mass of the people attributed the outbreak to the fact that the authorities buried filth in trenches close to their tents.... It is not to be wondered at that an ignorant and terror stricken multitude should have seized on the chief feature of the arrangements as the cause of all their troubles.

It was claimed that pilgrims viewed the epidemic as divine retribution by the goddess Kali, in whose hands they had hitherto placed their fate.[51] Such an interpretation is borne out by opposition to the regulation of internal pilgrimages in the Indian press. The Bengali newspaper, the *Hindoo Patriot*, for example, declared that 'any interference in them would be felt as a great hardship by the people' and supported J. M. Cuningham in his opposition to those who implicated pilgrimages in the spread of cholera.[52]

Fear of provoking civil unrest through heavy-handed intervention in the lives of Indians also lay behind the Indian government's increasing opposition to the use of quarantine and *cordons sanitaires.* On this issue, for a variety of medical and practical reasons, the majority of medical officers were at one with government. Advocates of the atmospheric theory of cholera dissemination associated with Bryden, and of Snow's waterborne theory, agreed that there was no medical logic in quarantine and thought it unnecessarily damaging to trade. Some also had humanitarian objections to the use of custodial sanitary measures. The Sanitary Commissioner of the Punjab, for instance, was unable to find words 'sufficiently strong' to express his disapproval of the forcible removal of the sick from their homes to hospital during a cholera epidemic in the province in 1872.[53]

Such measures appear to have been common practice in India in the years following the severe cholera outbreak of 1861; cantonment authorities being especially concerned to prevent the disease spreading among troops in the light of the Mutiny.[54] But, by 1870, the government was in a position to reflect on the factors which had led to the Mutiny and considered it politic, for reasons of public order, to discontinue *cordons sanitaires.* Colonial administrators were also concerned not to provide a precedent for custodial action at a time when they were being pressed on the issue of maritime quarantine. Yet, in 1873, three years after the resolution on *cordons sanitaires,* there were still several cantonment authorities that had not abandoned the practice, and as late as 1877, there were reports of quarantines being established against cholera at several military stations in Madras.[55] Indians wishing to enter cordoned towns were sometimes detained for up to ten days.

In opposition to *cordons sanitaires,* the Sanitary Commissioner, J. M. Cuningham, drew attention to the fact that no evidence had been produced to show that such measures were effective. 'The whole history of the epidemic', he argued, 'point[ed] to the danger of locality' and the only sensible response was the evacuation of troops to places thought to be free from cholera.[56] The government's favoured strategy against cholera was preventive action in the form of 'general sanitation', or 'practical sanitary action' as it was sometimes known. 'Cholera', wrote Cuningham, 'is to be dealt with on the same general principle as all other diseases.... Every sanitary defect must be sought out and, as far as possible remedied. [Cholera] is favoured by filth, overcrowding and every other condition adverse to health.'[57]

The responsibility for public health, in Cuningham's view, lay with individual municipalities and cantonment authorities. 'There can be no question', he advised government in 1873,

> that the municipalities must form the centres from which education in sanitary matters should spread among the people, and there is no more important duty for the Sanitary Commissioners to discharge than that of encouraging ... and creating the desire for sanitary improvements.[58]

This was an important departure, for it was now clearly recognized that the success of sanitary measures lay in cooperation with the indigenous population. The emphasis on education, of course, was also a means of transferring responsibility for sanitation onto the municipalities and the people themselves.

Cuningham knew that the epidemiological evidence regarding cholera was still very much open to interpretation. Investigations in Britain and India seemed to implicate the water supply in outbreaks of cholera, but there were counter-instances and, until such time as a causal organism was identified, evidence for the waterborne theory remained purely circumstantial.[59] While uncertainty remained it was possible to counter Snow's waterborne theory by an appeal to some other scientific authority.

With Bryden coming under increasing criticism, the Government of India cast its eyes abroad, as if to gain impartial vindication of its stance on cholera causation. It found a champion in the German hygienist Max von Pettenkofer whose 'sub-soil water' theory of cholera causation had already achieved widespread international recognition. Pettenkofer's theory did allow for the communicability of a hypothetical cholera 'germ', but placed most emphasis on the local factors thought to be necessary for its propagation. The most important of these factors was the presence of a porous soil and abnormally high levels of ground water.[60] Pettenkofer's preoccupation with locality and with environmental factors was well-suited to the Indian context. Cuningham also saw that, if it were shown to be correct, Pettenkofer's theory would place Indian sanitary practice on firmer foundations. The government's use of scientific expertise, then, was highly selective: aetiological positions did not so much determine, as provide a justification for, existing sanitary policies.[61]

Thus, in 1870 a scheme for the registration of sub-soil water levels was instituted in Madras, being extended to other provinces the following year.[62] However, the results of sub-soil water registration fell short of vindicating Pettenkofer. The first year of registration had been one which was 'unfortunately immune' from disease, so no significant correlation could be established.[63] Nevertheless, the government persisted with its programme, insisting that while Pettenkofer's theory had not been proved it had not yet been disproved either.[64] Provincial sanitary commissioners, many of whom had already been converted to the waterborne theory, were reluctant to continue the scheme. 'It is not clear', commented A. C. Lyall, Secretary of the Government of India, in 1874,

> on what grounds the Sanitary Commissioner for Bengal considers it unnecessary to continue ... the sub-soil water registration. It is now generally admitted that local conditions are intimately concerned with the presence or absence of cholera.... Variations in sub-soil water level should continue to be registered on an improved basis.[65]

But by 1875 the registration scheme was becoming an embarrassment to the government. Its arch critic DeRenzy had the 'honour to report' that 'the observations on sub-soil water level made to test Professor Pettenkofer's theory ... have not led to any clear or decisive results'.[66] There was also opposition to Pettenkofer from medical men outside the Sanitary Department, though limited sources make it impossible to gauge accurately its extent. The *Indian Medical Gazette,* which claimed to represent medical opinion in India, begged Pettenkofer 'before he again attempt[ed] to lay down the law regarding the diffusion of cholera in India ... to consult authorities who can give him reliable information on the subject'.[67]

It was understandable that medical men in India would have felt devalued as a result of their government's decision to consult a foreign 'expert'. Moreover, the IMS had long valued experience of conditions in India over and above theoretical speculation. The *coup de grâce* was delivered to sub-soil water registration by the Army Sanitary Commission in 1879. It noted that registration had failed to produce any significant results and that 'no general theory' could account for the incidence of cholera in different parts of India.[68]

Statistical epidemiology formed by far the greatest part of the government's 'enquiry' into cholera. Yet related questions, such as the existence or identity of a causal organism, could not be entirely ignored. Most of the research undertaken by IMS officers in this regard was reactive and generally negative in character, its chief purpose being to disprove the existence of a specific pathogen. The only systematic investigations carried out to test the 'germ' hypothesis were those undertaken by D. D. Cunningham of the IMS and T. R. Lewis of the Army Medical Department. They were appointed Special Scientific Assistants to Cuningham in 1874, though both had been working on cholera for some years.[69] Of particular importance was the question of whether certain micro-organisms found in human blood in conjunction with certain diseases were causal agents or merely 'epiphenomena', bodies which appeared to increase as a *consequence* of disease. Lewis concluded that such organisms had no causal relationship to cholera and were 'not uncommonly ... associated with no physical disturbance of the normal condition'. That Lewis understood the wider significance of his work is clear from his comment that

> should the views now commonly advanced [on the existence of pathogenic micro-organisms] prove to be correct, the theory and practice of medicine would be radically affected, and possibly the future action of the state with regard to disease be materially modified.[70]

In order to place the Indian cholera debates in context, it is useful to consider how the views of the various parties were reported in the British medical press. As early as 1870, the *Lancet* expressed an unfavourable opinion of Bryden's theory, arguing that human intercourse was of 'primary importance' in the diffusion of cholera.[71] The following year it threw its weight solidly behind DeRenzy, recommending his *Report on the Sanitary Administration of the Punjab*. 'It is so clearly written', wrote the journal's editor, 'that we have occasion to do little other than strictly follow it.... We regard it as an uncommonly good one.'[72] Cuningham's *Report on the Cholera Epidemic of 1872* was not so well received. 'Its conclusions', claimed the *Lancet*, 'are at variance with all the prevalent doctrines, and the author does not hesitate to combat every hypothesis that has been advanced regarding the nature, origin and development of epidemic cholera.'[73]

Neither did Cuningham's address to the Royal Medical and Chirurgical Society in London in 1874 ingratiate him with the metropolitan profession. His manner, protested a correspondent to the *British Medical Journal*, had been 'arrogant' and 'dismissive of all cholera research in Britain over the last 100 years'.[74] 'Dr Cuningham', wrote the editor of the *Lancet*,

> spoke of contagion as if it were a self-operative Frankenstein giving laws to itself.... Hardly less extraordinary was the fallacy that because India was the home of cholera ... observations made there had a pre-eminent advantage over observations conducted elsewhere.[75]

The respected physician Dr Netten Radcliffe had a similar view of Cuningham's work. 'The contagion of which Dr Cuningham spoke', he maintained, 'was not the contagion understood in this country; the water-theory had not the faintest resemblance to what is meant here.... Dr Cuningham judged of the contagion of cholera as if were operative in the same way as smallpox.'[76]

By narrowing down all notions of 'contagion' in this way, Cuningham hoped to place official theory beyond falsification.[77] So long as Cuningham continued to contrast cholera with smallpox he was able to hold up its 'preference' for certain localities and the absence of cases among those who tended the sick, as evidence against its communicability.

The Cholera Commissions

Thus throughout the 1870s official medical doctrine in India diverged increasingly from medical opinion in Britain. This was still the case for much of the 1880s, although, from the middle of the decade, following Robert Koch's claim to have discovered an organism causing cholera, there began a major shift in the official Indian position on cholera and in the means by which the disease was investigated. Robert Koch (1843–1910) and the German Cholera Commission arrived in Calcutta in December 1883. The Commission had already spent several months making clinical examinations of cholera patients in Egypt. There it had identified vast quantities of a particular bacterium in the intestines of persons suffering from cholera, but it was by no means clear whether these organisms bore any causal relation to the disease.[78]

In Calcutta the Commission was the guest of J. M. Cuningham, in his last year as Sanitary Commissioner. The Commission was provided with a small laboratory and such equipment as the Calcutta Medical College could afford.[79] In February, after isolating the 'Egyptian' bacillus from a water tank in Calcutta, the Commission announced that they had discovered the causal organism of cholera. Several cases of the disease had very recently occurred among people who regularly drew their drinking water from the tank.[80] Koch's assertion contradicted everything Cuningham and his superiors held to be true of cholera; moreover, his claims were made on the basis of evidence gathered in India itself. The isolation of the cholera bacillus called into question Cuningham's professional competence and threatened to undermine the theoretical basis of the government's sanitary policy. This memorandum by Surgeon-General Fayrer, President of the India Office Medical Board, is one of the clearest statements of the official reaction to Koch's claims:

> the doctrine of contagion ... is still maintained by many influential authorities on the Continent and here; the former loudly insisting on quarantine and charging us with conniving at the introduction of cholera to Europe, rather than interfere with our own mercantile interests.... That a bacillus in association with cholera has been detected there need be no question ... but that the cause of cholera has been discovered any more than it was before ... I believe to be a dangerous and unverifiable statement, inasmuch as it will tend to emphasize the views of contagion and the importance of quarantine already so much insisted on.[81]

Fayrer's memorandum draws attention to one of the chief weaknesses of Koch's argument. Koch had successfully demonstrated the existence of the 'comma bacillus' and its association with cholera, but he had not proven conclusively that it was the cause and not merely a consequence of the disease. Koch's theory rested solely on his ability to show that large numbers of the bacillus were present in the intestines of an infected person, and absent from persons free from infection. Another weak link in Koch's theory was his inability to reproduce the disease in animals, though, on this score, he was able to draw analogies with other diseases widely supposed to be 'contagious', like leprosy and typhoid.[82] Nevertheless, Koch's assertions were taken sufficiently seriously by the British government to warrant the formation of a team of researchers to investigate his findings. The English Cholera Commission, which comprised the distinguished London-based bacteriologists Edward Klein and Heneage Gibbes, was to work in conjunction with the Sanitary Department, but remain free from official interference. The two doctors received Rs 400 per month in payment for their services, up to Rs 50 for expenditure on scientific equipment, and free passage on board a P. & O. steamer to Bombay.[83]

Much to the satisfaction of both the British and Indian governments, the commission concluded that 'the comma bacillus in acute typical cases of cholera [was] by no means present in such numbers and with such frequency as to justify Koch's statement that the ileum contains almost a pure cultivation of cholera bacilli'.[84] These conclusions cast doubt on the strongest part of Koch's thesis – his presence/absence argument. According to E. R. Lankester in a letter to *The Times* in November 1884, Koch stood 'self-condemned'. He had not reproduced the disease in man or animal, and yet he had 'staked his reputation on the dogmatic assertion that the comma bacillus is the cause of cholera'.[85]

From Locality to Laboratory

But, for the most part, Koch's auditors accepted his claim that the comma bacillus was the causal organism of cholera. As Coleman puts it, 'the evidence [by analogy with other diseases] was persuasive if not conclusive'.[86] At the same time, it appeared to the Government of India that the controversy would be resolved in the laboratory rather than on the basis of purely epidemiological evidence. It was this realization that prompted it to improve facilities for medical research in India. The inadequacy of existing provisions had been highlighted by the visit of the English Cholera Commission, which had conducted its enquiry in a makeshift laboratory in the Calcutta Medical College.[87]

In December 1884, in accordance with a directive from the India Office, the Government of India sanctioned, at a cost of Rs 15,000, the construction in Calcutta of India's first medical laboratory. It realized that the enquiry into cholera might 'extend over a considerable period of time'.[88] In his capacity as Special Scientific Assistant to the Sanitary Commissioner, D. D. Cunningham was appointed Director of the laboratory, a post he would hold in conjunction with his professorship of physiology at the Calcutta Medical College. With his track record of opposition to cholera 'contagion', Cunningham, another Edinburgh graduate, was the obvious choice.[89] These developments were a clear departure from the statistical epidemiology of the 1860s and 1870s. Increasingly, the attempts of senior IMS officers to 'save the phenomena' of local causation led them into the unfamiliar world of bacteriology. Few IMS officers had experience of microscopical research and even fewer had been trained in bacteriological techniques.

It was no mere coincidence that the year of Koch's discovery saw the foundation of India's first journal of medical research. The first editor of *Scientific Memoirs by Medical Officers of the Army of India* was

Surgeon-General B. Simpson (1831–1923), Cuningham's successor as Sanitary Commissioner. The first edition of *Scientific Memoirs* carried an article by D. D. Cunningham, 'On the relation of cholera to schizomycete organisms', which purported to demonstrate that bacilli in the intestine of cholera patients might assume several forms, varying according to temperature, acidity and so on. Cunningham claimed that this discovery undermined Koch's claim to have identified a fixed species of bacillus in association with cholera. Cunningham was well aware that he had arrived at a conclusion 'in direct conflict with the majority of pathological bacteriologists'.[90]

Three years later, Cunningham continued his assault upon Koch, arguing that the comma bacillus was a comparatively 'feeble' organism unable to survive for long outside the human body. If this did not disprove Koch's theory, it seemed to place a great deal of emphasis on the environment necessary for the generation of cholera. 'If the choleraic commas really be the essential cause of the disease', he argued, 'then the facts would lead us to regard their agency in the production of epidemics as entirely subordinate to... local conditions.'[91] In 1889 Cunningham reiterated his belief that 'no contagionist theory will account for the phenomena of epidemic diffusion' and that Pettenkofer was correct in insisting on 'the primacy of local conditions'.[92]

By 1894 Cunningham had conceded that the comma bacillus was, in fact, a distinct organism associated with the 'choleraic condition', but refused to acknowledge that it was the sole, 'efficient' cause of the disease. Cunningham now advocated a modified version of Pettenkofer's theory which allowed for the action of 'two distinct poisons' – one manufactured in the intestinal tract, the other in the outside environment. Certain 'environmental' factors – particularly humidity – gave rise to a 'cholera poison' which was capable of producing the disease in an individual only if comma bacilli were present. If no comma bacilli were present, exposure to the 'cholera poison' would result in nothing more than mild ptomaine poisoning.[93] In this way Cunningham was able to square growing international acceptance of the role of the comma bacilli with the Government of India's insistence on the importance of local factors in the production of cholera. It was a theory which was also capable of explaining the limited success of the cholera inoculation developed by Waldemar Haffkine, while preserving a central role for 'general sanitation'.[94]

The fact that most discussion of the cholera controversy was limited to official journals and reports makes it difficult to generalize about the extent to which Koch's findings were accepted by the IMS as a whole. Editorial statements in the *Indian Medical Gazette* at the time when Koch's discovery was first made public display a certain sympathy with Koch's endeavours but acknowledge that the matter was still far from resolved.[95] But the conclusions of the English Cholera Commission tilted the balance decisively against Koch. 'That Dr Koch has certainly not proved that the comma bacillus ... is the [cause of cholera] must now be regarded as clear', insisted the *Gazette,* 'indeed his supporters have now withdrawn so far from their position as to admit this; and they now simply allege its diagnostic importance.'[96]

In order to assess to what extent these pronouncements were representative of the views of the British profession as a whole it is perhaps wise to consider the personal viewpoint of the journal's editor, Kenneth MacLeod. MacLeod, editor of the *Indian Medical Gazette* from 1871 to 1892, was a public advocate of the waterborne theory and critical of Pettenkofer, Bryden and the Government of India. In his assessment of Pettenkofer's work, MacLeod had shown himself hostile to interference from 'outsiders' who presumed to understand cholera better than the IMS itself. This may partly explain his lukewarm reception of Koch's thesis. Nevertheless, as editor of the *IMG* and as a distinguished medical man in his own right, MacLeod's views would have been influential in shaping medical opinion in India.[97]

But it was only after 1893, following Georg Gaffky's analysis of the Hamburg cholera epidemic the previous year, that Koch's theory came to command almost universal assent among medical men in Europe. Gaffky had established the critical role of drinking water in the spread of the epidemic, providing firm epidemiological evidence to support Koch's hypothesis.[98] But official acceptance of Koch's theory in Germany, as Richard Evans has shown, owed as much to political factors as to the force of scientific logic.[99] At the same time, Koch actually opposed maritime quarantine – it was his belief that cholera invariably spread to Europe overland from India. This made Koch's theory attractive to the British government and, increasingly, to the other European powers whose traffic in the Mediterranean and through the Suez Canal had increased markedly in the 1880s and 1890s.

These developments convinced most European medical men of the validity or, at least, the utility of Koch's theory.[100] Koch's theory also received confirmation from epidemiological evidence obtained in India.[101] But Cunningham clung to his position that the comma bacillus had a 'definite causal relation' to cholera only under certain conditions within the intestinal tract. These intestinal conditions were themselves, in certain circumstances, influenced by the 'external environment'.[102] The breadth and complexity of Pettenkofer's theory provided the basis for compromise: in its modified form, it seemed to allow for both the existence of a specific causal organism and for the influence of certain environmental factors.

Increasingly, the question became one of emphasis. As Ira Klein puts it, in the mid-1890s 'it was no longer fashionable to deny completely the germ theory of disease'.[103] But within this new framework there was still disagreement over the media in which the cholera bacillus was spread, and particularly over the measures required to prevent it. These disagreements are best illustrated by the dispute between W. A. Roe – Sanitary Commissioner for the Punjab – and W. R. Rice – Sanitary Commissioner with the Government of India – over measures to arrest the disease. Roe, a microbiologist, maintained that preventive measures should be focused specifically on the bacillus' chief mode of transmission – the water supply. Rice, however, believed that there were many sources of infection and continued to favour a broad, non-exclusive approach to sanitation.[104]

By the early twentieth century these conflicts had been largely resolved, with wide agreement among medical men in India on the utility of specific measures against cholera, but as merely one part of a more general sanitary programme.[105] No longer was there thought to be any fundamental contradiction between the aims of research scientists and those who struggled on a day-to-day basis with practical sanitation. The identity of cholera had clearly been transformed by the growing importance of laboratory diagnosis but this had been a very gradual process, in which the cholera pathogen had been integrated within a pre-existing aetiological framework.

Conclusion

The politics of cholera in nineteenth-century India demonstrate to a striking degree the importance of the geographical identity of the disease. Though global in its dissemination, cholera never lost its association with India, though this was construed in very different ways. Most people in nineteenth-century Europe regarded cholera as 'Asiatic' in the sense of an alien invader probably originating in India. But the Government of India, and many of those in the IMS, portrayed cholera in South Asia as essentially different from the disease in Europe. They denied that Indian cholera had ever been transmitted outside the usual 'epidemic areas', which were said to be bounded by the limits of the monsoon winds. Such notions were firmly in keeping with the traditional British conception of India as epidemiologically unique but the emphasis on locality and atmosphere was also politically convenient in that it was congruent with a *laissez-faire* sanitary policy. It provided a theoretical justification for opposition to large sanitary engineering works, such as those advocated by the government's critics, and to *cordons sanitaires* and other potentially dangerous forms of intervention in Indian society. In this sense cholera theory and the question of locality lay at the heart of debates about how to govern India and about the nature of imperial responsibilities.

Resistance to the universalizing claims of metropolitan medicine contributed to the increasing perception of India as a scientific backwater and a sanitary pariah. British India's isolation did not end until the 1890s when, after attempting to compete with metropolitan science on its own terms, its government was forced into line with international medical opinion. Yet cholera did not cease to be regarded as a predominantly Asian disease. At the turn of the century, by which time cholera had been stamped out in most European countries through improvements in sanitation and water supplies, the disease continued to ravage India and other poorer areas of the world. Colonial governments lacked both the will and the resources to take effective action. Though manifestly a disease of poverty, cholera was still widely regarded as one of place.

Notes

I am grateful to members of the audience at the Wellcome Syposium 'Tropical Medicine Before Manson' who commented on an earlier draft of this essay. A somewhat different version appears as chapter 4 of M. Harrison, *Public Health in British India: Anglo-Indian Preventive Medicine, 1859–1914* (Cambridge: Cambridge University Press, 1994).

1. E. Le Roy Ladurie, 'A concept: The unification of the globe by disease', in his *The Mind and Method of the Historian* (Brighton: Harvester, 1983), 28–83.
2. On the spread of epidemic cholera in and from India, see D. Arnold, 'Cholera morality in British India, 1817–1947', in T. Dyson (ed.), *India's Historical Demography: Studies in Famine, Disease, and Society* (London: Curzon Press, 1989), 261–84; *idem,* 'The Indian Ocean as a disease zone, 1500–1950', *South Asia,* 14 (1991), 1–22.
3. On the collective international response to cholera, see N. E. Goodman, *International Health Organisations and their Work* (London: Churchill, 1952); N. Howard-Jones, *The Scientific Background of the International Sanitary Conferences, 1851–1938* (Geneva: WHO, 1975).
4. With the exception of the British and Government of India delegates,

the conferences from 1866 agreed that cholera was communicated in the discharges of infected persons mingling with water. They did not believe that the disease was communicable from person to person in the same way as smallpox.

5. On the emergence of a distinctive medical tradition in British India see M. Harrison, 'Tropical medicine in nineteenth-century India', *British Journal for the History of Science,* 25 (1992), 299–318, and *op. cit.* (notes intro.), Ch. 2.
6. The perception of India as a distinctive disease environment is discussed at length in M. Harrison, '"The tender frame of man": Climatic anxiety and racial difference in British India and the West Indies, 1760–1860', *Bulletin of the History of Medicine* (forthcoming).
7. See I. Klein, 'Cholera theory and treatment in nineteenth-century India', *Journal of Indian History,* 58 (1980), 35–51; D. Arnold, 'Cholera and colonialism in British India', *Past and Present,* 113 (1986), 118–51.
8. M. Harrison, 'Quarantine, pilgrimage, and colonial trade: India 1866–1900', *Indian Economic and Social History Review,* 29 (1992), 117–44. The epidemiological dimension of the Hadj is also discussed in J. Baldry, 'The Ottoman quarantine station on Kamaran island 1882–1914', *Studies in the History of Medicine,* 2 (1978), 18–19; Howard-Jones, *op. cit.* (note 3), N. E. Gallagher, *Medicine and Power in Tunisia, 1780–1900* (Cambridge: Cambridge University Press, 1983).
9. François Delaporte, *Disease and Civilization: The Cholera in Paris, 1832* (Cambridge, Mass.: MIT Press, 1986). I am grateful to Michael Worboys for letting me read his unpublished manuscript: 'Medical History and the Germ Theory of Disease'.
10. C. E. Rosenberg, 'Disease in history: Frames and framers', *The Milbank Quarterly,* 67 (1989) 1–15.
11. A. Cunningham, 'Transforming plague: The laboratory and the identity of infectious disease', in A. R. Cunningham and P. Williams, *The Laboratory Revolution in Medicine* (Cambridge: Cambridge University Press, 1992), 209–44.
12. B. Latour, *The Pasteurization of France* (London: Harvard University Press, 1988).
13. For a critique of Latour's work see S. Sturdy, 'The germs of a new Enlightenment', *Studies in the History and Philosophy of Science,* 22 (1991), 163–73.
14. See E. H. Ackerknecht, 'Anticontagionism between 1821 and 1861', *Bulletin of the History of Medicine,* 22 (1948), 561–93; R. J. Morris, *Cholera 1832: The Social Response to an Epidemic* (London: Croom Helm, 1976).
15. M. Pelling, *Cholera, Fever, and English Medicine, 1825–1865* (Oxford: Oxford University Press, 1978); M. Durey, *The Return of the Plague: British Society and the Cholera 1831–2* (Dublin: Gill and MacMillan, 1979); G. P. Parsons, 'The British medical profession

and contagion theory: Peurperal fever as a case study, 1830–1860', *Medical History,* 22 (1978), 138–50; R. Cooter, 'Anticontagionism and history's medical record', in P. Wright and A. Treacher (eds), *The Problem of Medical Knowledge* (Edinburgh: Edinburgh University Press, 1982), 87–108.

16. D. G. Crawford, *Roll of the Indian Medical Service* (London: Thacker, 1933) 154 and *Lancet* obituary, ii (1880), 915–16.
17. J. L. Bryden, *Cholera Epidemics of Recent Years Viewed in Relation to Former Epidemics: A Record of Cholera in the Bengal Presidency from 1817 to 1872* (Calcutta: Superintendent of Government Press, 1874), 1. See also Bryden's *Epidemic Cholera in Bengal* (Calcutta: Superintendent of Government Press, 1869); *Lancet,* i (1870), 209.
18. L. J. Jordanova, 'Earth science and environmental medicine: The synthesis of the late Enlightenment', in L. J. Jordanova and R. Porter (eds), *Images of the Earth: Essays in the History of the Environmental Sciences* (Cambridge: British Society for the History of Science, 1979), 122; K. Thomas, *Man and the Natural World: Changing Attitudes in England 1500–1800* (London: Penguin, 1983), 31.
19. Jordanova, 'Earth science and environmental medicine' *op. cit.,* (note 18), 135.
20. J. L. Bryden, *The Cholera History of 1875 and 1876* (Calcutta: Superintendent of Government Press, 1878), 308–13.
21. See D. Kumar, 'The evolution of colonial science in India: Natural history and the East India Company', in J. M. MacKenzie (ed.) *Imperialism and the Natural World* (Manchester: Manchester University Press, 1990), 51–66.
22. J. M. Eyler, 'The conceptual origins of William Farr's epidemiology: Numerical methods and social thought in the 1830s', in A. M. Lilienfeld (ed.), *Times, Places and Persons: Aspects of the History of Epidemiology* (Baltimore: Johns Hopkins University Press, 1980), 11–13.
23. See: J. L. Bryden's *Vital Statistics of the Bengal Presidency* (Calcutta: Superintendent of Government Press, 1866–79).
24. *Lancet* obituary of Bryden, ii (1880), 913–16. Farr was somewhat more cautious in making claims about the predictive value of his work than Bryden: Eyler, *op. cit.* (note 22), 8–9.
25. *British Medical Journal* (hereafter *BMJ*), 15 August, 1868, 173.
26. Bryden quoted in *Lancet,* 5 February, 1870, 209.
27. *Ibid.,* 81.
28. *Lancet,* i (1905), 122; Crawford, *op. cit.* (note 16), 138. Cuningham graduated four years before Bryden.
29. Klein, *op. cit.* (note 7), 38.
30. India Office Records (hereafter IOR) P/674. Government of India (hereafter GOI), (Sanitary), DeRenzy to Secretary to GOI, 13 September, 1871. DeRenzy's emphasis on sanitary measures designed to protect the water supply is clearly stated in *Report of the Sanitary*

Commissioner of the Punjab (1868), 25, 39. DeRenzy advocated a closed-pipe water supply for towns and military cantonments.

31. E. A. Parkes, *A Manual of Practical Hygiene* (London: Churchill, 1864), 21–4, 36, 47–8. However, no causal organism had yet been identified in the case of cholera and there existed considerable uncertainty in Britain at this time as to the exact nature of the threat posed by impure water. See C. Hamlin, 'Politics and germ theories in Victorian Britain: The metropolitan water commissions of 1867–9 and 1892–3', in R. MacLeod (ed.), *Government and Expertise: Specialists, Administrators and Professionals, 1860–1919* (Cambridge: Cambridge University Press, 1988), 110–27.
32. IOR P/674. GOI (Sanitary), DeRenzy to Sec. to GOI, 13 September, 1871.
33. GOI (Sanitary), DeRenzy to Sec. to GOI, 13 September, 1871: 'Dr Bryden's theory is merely the old one professing to rest on a statistical basis and until now there were few Indian Medical Officers who disagreed with or dissented from it.'
34. GOI (Sanitary), DeRenzy to Sec. to GOI, 13 September, 1871, citing Cuningham's sanitary report for 1870.
35. IOR P/674. GOI (Sanitary), Sec. to GOI to Sec. to Punjab government, No. 38, 23 January, 1872.
36. *Indian Public Opinion and Punjab Times,* 29 March, 1870.
37. IOR P/434/45. GOI (Sanitary), Sec. to GOB to Sec. to GOI, No. 1221, 6 April, 1870.
38. IOR P/1338. GOI (Sanitary), memo. of Army Sanitary Commission (hereafter ASC) on the report of the Sanitary Commission of the North-West Provinces and Oudh (hereafter NWP & O) for 1877, No. 2, November 1879.
39. IOR P/1498. GOI (Sanitary), memo. of ASC on report of Sanitary Commission for Bengal for 1878, No. 17, January 1880.
40. *Indian Medical Gazette* (hereafter *IMG*), June 1872, 186.
41. *IMG,* October 1873, 265.
42. R. Ramasubban, 'Imperial health in British India', in R. MacLeod and M. Lewis (eds), *Disease, Medicine, and Empire: Perspectives on Western Medicine and the Experience of European Expansion* (London: Routledge, 1988), 41.
43. F. Nightingale, *Life or Death in India? A Paper read at the meeting of the National Association for the Promotion of Social Science, Norwich, 1873,* (London: NAPSS, 1873), 15.
44. Viscount Mersey, *The Viceroys and Governors-General of India 1757–1947* (London: Murray, 1949), 82–7.
45. R. J. Moore, *Liberalism and Indian Politics* (London: Arnold, 1966), 15. The administration of India had become decentralized in 1861, when local legislatures were set up for the first time in Madras, Bombay and Bengal. Other legislatures were established subsequently under powers conferred by this Act.

46. R. Ramasubban, *Public Health and Medical Research: Their Origins under the Impact of British Colonial Policy* (Stockholm: SAREC, 1982), 22–3.
47. Crawford, *op. cit.* (note 16), 105. Murray's best known works were *Topography of Meerut* (1839) and *Topography of Fatehpur Sikri* (1835). His first treatise on cholera was not published until 1869, two years after the epidemic.
48. 'Report on the Cholera of 1867' in *Report of the Sanitary Commissioner with the Government of India* (hereafter *SCGI*), (1867), 134–5.
49. J. Murray, *Report on the Treatment of Epidemic Cholera* (Calcutta: Superintendent of Government Press, 1869), 7.
50. Ramasubban, *op. cit.* (note 46), 22. But, though Murray's plan for 'pilgrim stations' *en route* to religious fairs found little favour with the government, sanitary provisions continued to be made at places of pilgrimage themselves. See, for example, I. J. Ranking, *Madras Fairs and Festivals* (Madras: 1868).
51. *Report on the Cholera Epidemic of 1867 in Northern India* (Calcutta: Superintendent of Government Press, 1867), 17–18.
52. *Hindoo Patriot,* 28 July, 1879.
53. IOR P/525. GOI (Sanitary), DeRenzy to Sec. to Punjab government, 5 June, 1873. Where sanitary measures impinged on indigenous ways of life, DeRenzy favoured the use of indigenous personnel, even practitioners of indigenous medicine. However, the employment of *vaids* and *hakims* was stubbornly resisted by other members of the medical profession, and in the Punjab the system was brought to an end in the 1880s. See J. C. Hume, 'Rival traditions: Western medicine and Yunan-i Tibb in the Punjab, 1849–1889', *Bulletin of the History of Medicine,* 51 (1977), 214–31; *idem,* 'Colonialism and sanitary medicine: The development of preventive health policy in the Punjab, 1860–1900', *Modern Asian Studies,* 20 (1986), 703–24.
54. The commission which investigated the cholera epidemic of 1861 expressed the view that cholera was communicated by 'human intercourse' and recommended the isolation of sick troops from their healthy counterparts. The Commission's recommendations appear to have been followed in most cantonments and in some civilian areas like the city of Bombay: *Proceedings of the Sanitary Commissioner for Bombay* (1866), 2, 43–9. The Sanitary Commissioner of Bombay also attempted, without success, to persuade railway companies to prohibit persons suffering from cholera from using their trains: *Proceedings of the Sanitary Commisioner for Bombay* (1867), 238.
55. *Indian Public Opinion and Punjab Times,* 6 January, 1877.
56. *SCGI* (1875), 157–8.
57. *SCGI* (1877), 81. See also J. M. Cuningham, *Cholera: What can the State do to prevent it?* (Calcutta: Superintendent of Government Press, 1884).

58. IOR P/525. GOI (Sanitary), Cuningham to Sec. to GOI, 18 August, 1873.
59. Different conclusions on the spread of cholera could be drawn from the same epidemiological data: H. Letheby, 'Report on the sanitary condition of the city of London', quoted in *BMJ,* 22 February, 1868, 173; William Farr's 'Report on the Cholera Epidemic of 1866', in *BMJ,* 15 August, 1868, 169.
60. Howard-Jones, *op. cit.* (note 3), 22–34.
61. As in Britain: see Hamlin, *op. cit.* (note 31).
62. IOR P/434/45. GOI (Sanitary), No. 283, Sanitary Commissioner of Madras to Sec. to GOI, 8 March, 1870.
63. *SCGI* (1871), 73.
64. *SCGI* (1872), 35.
65. IOR P/525. GOI (Sanitary), Sec. to GOI to Sec. to Government of Bengal (Judicial Dept.), 22 December, 1874.
66. IOR P/525. GOI (Sanitary), DeRenzy to Sec. to Punjab government, 11 May, 1875.
67. *IMG,* June 1872, 186.
68. IOR P/1003. GOI (Sanitary), memo. of ASC on report of the Sanitary Commisioner of Bengal for 1877.
69. *SCGI* (1874), 42–3.
70. T. R. Lewis, 'The microscopic organisms found in the blood of man and animals and their relation to disease', in *SCGI* (1877), 157–8. Lewis quoted Charles Murchison, the renowned British expert on fever, in defence of his views, 185–6.
71. *Lancet,* 1 February, 1870, 209.
72. *Lancet,* 14 January, 1871, 52.
73. *Lancet,* 15 November, 1873, 707.
74. *BMJ,* 21 August, 1880, 234.
75. *Lancet,* 4 April, 1874, 482.
76. *Ibid.,* 477.
77. Essentially the same technique was used by both Southwood Smith and William Budd with respect to cholera theory in Britain, the former categorically opposing all notions of 'contagion', the latter, explaining the behaviour of epidemic disease by reference to smallpox. See Pelling, *op. cit.* (note 15), 50–79, 250–93.
78. W. Coleman, 'Koch's comma bacillus: The first year', *Bulletin of the History of Medicine,* 61 (1987), 315–42; T. D. Brock, *Robert Koch: A Life in Medicine and Bacteriology* (Madison: Science Tech. Publishers, 1988), 150–67.
79. Coleman, *op. cit.* (note 78), 324–5. The political implications of the Commission's visit are discussed more fully in Harrison, *op. cit.* (notes intro.), Ch. 8.
80. *SCGI* (1884), 159.
81. *Procs. Madras Sanitary Commissioner,* No. 42, 1884, memo. of 19 May, 1884 to all provincial governments.

82. Coleman, *op. cit.* (note 78), 327.
83. *Procs. Madras Sanitary Commissioner,* No. 42, 1884, Under–Sec. of State for India to GOI, 26 July, 1884.
84. *SCGI* (1884), 159.
85. *The Times,* 19 November, 1884.
86. Coleman, *op. cit.* (note 78), 337.
87. *SCGI* (1884), 160. There had, for some years, been complaints about the Government of India's neglect of medical research: e.g., see *IMG,* January 1882, 17.
88. IOR P/2708. GOI (Sanitary), Sec. to Government of Bengal to Sec. to GOI, 14 February, 1885.
89. IOR P/2708. GOI (Sanitary), Sec. to GOI to Sec. of State for India, 18 May, 1886. David Douglas Cunningham (1843–1914) was educated at Edinburgh and Munich, where he worked under Pettenkofer, then Professor of Hygiene. Cunningham joined the IMS in 1868, rising to the rank of surgeon-major at the time of his appointment to the directorship of the cholera laboratory and retiring, in 1892, as a brigade surgeon lieutenant-colonel with extra pension. In addition to numerous reports on cholera, he was the author, with T. R. Lewis, of 'Fungus disease in India', *Quain's Dictionary of Medicine* (1882) and *Physiological and Pathological Researches* (1888). See Crawford, *op. cit.* (note 16), 174.
90. D. D. Cunningham, 'On the relation of cholera to schizomycete organisms', *Scientific Memoirs of Medical Officers of the Government of India* (hereafter *Sci. Mems.*) (1884), 1–16.
91. *Idem.,* 'Results of examinations of old specimens of choleraic tissues', *Sci. Mems.* (1887), 1–11.
92. *Idem.,* 'Are choleraic bacilli really efficient in determining the diffusion of cholera?', *Sci. Mems.* (1889), 1–20.
93. *Idem.,* 'The results of continued study of various forms of comma bacillus occurring in Calcutta', *Sci. Mems.* (1894), 1–57.
94. Haffkine's inoculation was tested on a number of occasions in India in 1894, allegedly with a certain amount of success. See, for example, W. J. Simpson, *Cholera in Calcutta in 1894 and Anti-Choleraic Inoculation* (Calcutta: Superintendent of Government Press, 1894).
95. *IMG,* May 1884, 142.
96. *IMG,* May 1885, 115.
97. Kenneth MacLeod (1840–1922) held the post of Professor of Surgery and First Surgeon at Calcutta Medical College from 1879 to 1896. He was an active propagandist of a more interventionist approach to public health, being chairman of the Calcutta Health Society. See Crawford, *op. cit.* (note 16), *BMJ* obituary, ii (1922), 1246; *Lancet,* ii (1922), 1403, *Plarr's Lives of the Fellows of the Royal College of Surgeons of England* (1930), II, 8–9.
98. Coleman, *op. cit.* (note 78), 341.
99. R. J. Evans, *Death in Hamburg: Society and Politics in the Cholera*

Years 1830–1910 (Oxford: Oxford University Press, 1990). Koch's demand for strong state intervention against cholera accorded with the Imperial government's desire to impose its authority on the Federal States (270).

100. *BMJ*, 25 February, 1893, 429–30. There were, however, exceptions. See *BMJ*, 20 January, 1894, 120–22; C. Creighton, *A History of Epidemics in Britain*, 2 vols, (Cambridge: Cambridge University Press, 1891–4).
101. *SCGI* (1895), 181.
102. D. D. Cunningham, 'Choleraic and other commas: On the influence of certain conditions determining morphological variations in vibrionic organisms', *Sci. Mems.* (1897), 1–29.
103. Klein, *op. cit.* (note 7), 47.
104. *Ibid.*, 47–50.
105. See, for example, *Proceedings of the All-India Sanitary Conference, 1911* (Calcutta: Superintendent of Government Press, 1912), especially the presidential address, 1–2.

8

Tropical without the Tropics: The Turning-Point of Pastorian Medicine in North Africa

Anne Marie Moulin

This essay relates to two of my present interests: on the one hand, the history of the overseas Pasteur Institutes, and on the other, the perception of Arabic culture through colonial medicine in Mediterranean countries. I would like to suggest an answer to a question which haunts the discussions on the medicine of warm climates prior to 1880 and the Pastorian brand of tropical medicine.[1] Were they so very different, and how were they different? I will make the point that, if they were actually different, the Pastorians over-emphasized the difference by claiming a scientific revolution that swept away the past and marked the starting point of modern medicine.[2]

The emergence of tropical medicine at the end of the nineteenth century represented the emergence of a paradigm of medical research in which vector-transmitted diseases played a major role. The generic term 'parasite' included all living pathogens and referred to their biological dependence on the host organism. After a period of doubt, the protozoan plasmodium was identified by Laveran as the agent of malaria. Parasitology figured as an extension of microbiology in the Pastorian programme.

Nevertheless, the 'mosquito theory', put forward by Ross and Grassi in the 1890s, shattered the simplicity of the germ theory of disease and provided a new pattern of investigation in the natural foci of the disease. This theory singled out an additional link, the vector, in a causal chain of the disease which listed the following: germs or parasites, intermediate hosts or vectors, and virus reservoirs. It was hoped that vectors such as insects could be wiped out, that attenuated or killed vaccines could be produced, and, in short, that the era of scientifically-guided eradication had begun. Around 1900, parasitic infections or insect-borne diseases loomed large in the Pastorian programme of struggle against world-wide pestilences that completed the microbe-hunting initiated in the 1880s. From our contemporary vantage-point, we know how far away stood the eradication of parasitic diseases and how dramatically the environmental view forced its way back and made these earlier medical dreams appear unrealistic.

In the Maghreb, the medicine of warm climates was succeeded by Pastorian tropical medicine. For this Algeria stood as a somewhat extreme and strange case, its tropical character being debatable. 'Tropical'[3] was an elusive and polysemic designation, whose metaphoric meaning requires further analysis.

North Africa extends above the Tropic of Cancer and is located mainly in the temperate climatic zone. The region does not exhibit the attractive or repulsive characteristics of tropical countries: the Maghreb fostered neither the anthropological despair of the 'Sad Tropics',[4] nor the dreams roused by the 'Lands of Good Hope'.[5] However, so long as tropical coincided with colonial,[6] medicine in North Africa could legitimately be considered as 'para'-tropical at least, through numerous analogies with the tropical countries. This ambiguous status bore testimony to the complexity of factors underlying tropicality, among which the geographic feature was merely the most flamboyant. The metaphor of tropical indicated a general dependence on a harsh natural determinism among a population trapped by climatic and geographic conditions. In other words, tropical stood for poverty, and for physiological misery.

Medical thinking at the end of the nineteenth century, particularly in the French Pastorian school, focused on the tropical area. The tropics, the 'white man's grave',[7] were ill-famed for their insalubrity. Doctors accordingly viewed the tropics as the paramount stage for medical warfare and the ultimate triumph over disease. Western science would there achieve the demonstration of its excellence and superiority.

In the last decade of the nineteenth century, Algeria, Tunisia, and later Morocco, fell within the domain of 'tropical medicine' which was given, in the French context, the name of 'exotic pathology'. The French Society of Exotic Pathology[8] was founded by the Pastorians Laveran and Mesnil in 1908.[9] Félix Mesnil was the leading protozoologist of the Pasteur Institute in Paris and his role speaks eloquently of the importance of newly identified parasites in the realm of diseases.[10] Laveran was hardly a Pastorian. He achieved his main discovery, the description of the haematozoaire at Constantine in 1880, but he was incorporated into the Pastorian roll of honour in

1897 when he retired from the army and joined the institute, where he received a laboratory. The *Bulletin de Pathologie exotique,* still extant today, was planned as a compendium of modern knowledge on overseas diseases. 'Exotic pathology' included tropical infections and their North African variants.

Tropicality, as manifested in North Africa, for instance by the prevalence of malaria, the archetypal tropical disease, was not seen to be intrinsic to the region, but rather an historical accident linked to political decadence. Consequently, the medical history of North Africa, as viewed in the 1930s by French medics, is the history of a shift from a temporary and contingent pseudo-tropical state to the normal position of a prosperous and modern country through the vigorous changes brought about by colonization. But the discourse on tropical medicine had eclipsed another medical language that prevailed in the early years of colonization. This language, where North Africa was simply referred to as a 'hot country', bore scientific as well as anthropological differences: the natives were perceived differently. In the first generation, the indigenous peoples received a lot of attention regarding their hygiene and lifestyle, while in Pastorian times, they receded into the background as an element in the transmission of disease in nature. They became stigmatized as the virus reservoir and were treated theoretically and practically as such.

Medicine of Warm Climates Prior to 1880

The importance and prestige of the medical profession developed considerably during the early years of colonization in Algeria.[11] At the beginning of the conquest in 1830, doctors played only a modest role.[12] They were mainly military surgeons, known for their ability to heal wounds, put together broken bones and amputate limbs. Baron Dominique Larrey, the famous surgeon, shown at work on the battlefield in so many pictures of the imperial wars with a knife in his hand,[13] embodied this tradition. He had followed Bonaparte to Egypt in 1802. He participated in the first months of the Algiers campaign under King Louis Philippe and died on his way back to France. During the campaign, he was helped by a local barber-surgeon and is said to have been fully satisfied with his skill in amputating.[14] Surgeons followed the army with the baggage train.[15] They had poor equipment and received little attention from the administration. They sometimes had to provide their own horses, if these were stolen or killed.

Yet, the sanitary reports on the French army and early settlers sounded quite disastrous. The French fell less to Arab bullets than as prey to various fevers.[16] The turnover rate of soldiers in hospitals was amazing. In one year, in effect, the whole army went to hospital three times: there was a permanent rotation, due to dysenteric bouts in every season and relapsing fevers in summer. The fate of recently established settlers was no better. Their life was a 'continuous oblation to death'.[17]

Doctors responded to the situation by placing the new pathology in a familiar context, the epidemic constitution[18] as analysed by Hippocratic tradition.[19] Hippocrates provided the framework of thought most appropriate to disentangling the puzzle of poorly understood fevers and ailments.[20] The physician Périer, reporting on health matters in Algeria, relied on the eighteenth-century model formulated by Vicq d'Azyr,[21] in suggesting 'registers for observation data', when after 1842, health officers were appointed by the administration (the so-called 'Bureaux arabes') to take care of the Arab population.

Scholarly interest in the remains of the Romans (the alleged ancestors of the French) played an important role in the French mental appropriation of Algeria. Archaeology was summoned to support the image of a prosperous Roman province, with a large population, prior to the Beni Hilal invasion. The responsibility for the subsequent decline fell upon the civil and foreign wars that had devastated the cultivated lands and multiplied the stagnant waters which produced miasmatic diseases. A vigorous strategy of settlement alone would reverse the course of history and revive past prosperity. The eradication of fevers was linked to the settlement of Europeans on fertile land and meant, in the short term, the eviction of the former proprietors, whether sedentary farmers or nomadic tribes. Malaria was indistinguishable from the colonization question.

In the meantime, waiting for a return to the epidemic constitution of *Africa romana*, the main question, crucial for the future of the colony, was whether settlers could hope to acclimatize. Travellers and settlers crossed climatic barriers which contained natural hosts. The problem was how to conceive the cosmopolitan nature of the human species while admitting to variations in terms of local adaptation. The nature and annual course of infections narrowly depended on climatic factors, falling into the fundamental categories of hot/cold, dry/wet, shaping in a specific way the humoral 'framework' of the organism.[22] But there was a distinction involved in opposing cursed countries to European paradises. On the one hand, natives no doubt benefited from a generation-long adaptation to their environment. This natural acclimatization would be redefined by the Pastorians in terms of immunity to local diseases.[23] On the other hand, the comparative study of pathology between North Africa and Europe revealed an interesting balance between morbid species. Dysenteries and recurring fevers were more common in warm climates while infections of the chest, above all tuberculosis, were exacting a frightening toll in industrialized countries. Did this mean 'no pain, no gain'? During the early years of colonization, the native offered an apparent solution to the central issue of adaptation. That perception changed dramatically in the following generation, at the end of the ninteenth century, when the indigenes came to figure as the main potential danger, being seen as the reservoirs or transmitters of disease.

In the early years of the conquest of Algeria, it was proposed that, in order to avoid suffering, immigrants should undergo a process of progressive adaptation.[24] Why not organize periods of adjustment in intermediate places, such as the south of France before sending them to Algeria, or send the recruits into the hills before despatching them to the Algerian mountains? These measures would test individual capabilities and allow a prediction of the eventual outcome. Above all, *métissage,* or racial mixing, was highly prized as the best way of combining local adaptation with the alleged superiority of the invader.[25] Algeria was not the only case where unions with local wives were warmly recommended to the soldier-settlers dear to Marshall Bugeaud: in Indonesia and West Africa, too, the advantages of racial mixing were advanced, before the beginning of European female immigration encouraged sexual segregation. In Algeria, the Arabs also massively rejected 'interbreeding', although probably less absolutely than has generally been stated. Such a medical vision was optimistic and somewhat contemplative. Acclimatization was a natural process that could only be quickened by improvement in diet and lifestyle, borrowing mainly from the Algerians themselves. The role of food, so important in Hippocratic therapeutics,[26] and the influence of stress and overwork were illustrated by differences in the fatality rate between soldiers and officers.

For the troops, avoidance strategies were seen to be best – camping far from obvious foci of epidemics, or in the uplands.[27] Quarantines remained in favour. On these points, Western medicine converged with contagionist trends in the Arab medical tradition on the appropriate behaviour to be followed in times of epidemics. Although the topic was a matter of controversy, many scholars cited the *hadith* that permitted choosing a minor injury in order to avoid a greater one.[28]

Another feature of this colonial medicine is the importance of

Orientalism. Among the distinguished physicians of the time, the most famous was Dr Lucien Leclerc, well known for his history of Arab medicine,[29] which is still of interest today. He edited numerous treatises by Zahrawi, Razi, and also from the medical schools of North Africa, such as the Cairene scholar, Ibn Jazzar. Almost all issues of the *Gazette médicale d'Alger,* founded in 1856, offered a selection of papers commenting on aspects of Arab surgery or pharmacopoeia, drawn from the study of original manuscripts.

Interestingly, the Hippocratic connection offered a unique opportunity for dialogue with the surviving Arab medical tradition, but this opportunity was hardly perceived. On the basis of the genuine scholarly interest in Arabic traditions,[30] and the acknowledgement of common roots, a dialogue might have been initiated between the two medical cultures, which had in the past enjoyed alternate periods in favour and had never stopped interacting. This opportunity finally disappeared with the terrible insurrection of the 1870s, the 'années de braise', and the gap between the vanquished and the conquerors widened.[31]

Dr Emile Bertherand, the author of a well-documented study called *Medicine and Hygiene among the Arabs*[32] did not perceive the Hippocratic flavour of local medicine, the familiarity of the classification of hot and warm diseases and the treatments accordingly prescribed. He mocked the excessive use of cautery, forgetting the controversies in Renaissance times on this subject. One wonders from where he drew this sense of superiority. A thorough study of pharmacopoeia would have shown that *kina,* the ancestor of 'colonial' quinine, had figured prominently among the treatments for relapsing fevers.[33] Apart from the treatment of malaria, the medicine of warm climates did not abound in specific cures and magic bullets. Medical works, more advice than prescriptions, aimed at protecting soldiers and settlers from dangerous miasmas by encouraging the use of appropriate clothing, the moderate use of wine and spirits and sexual abstinence,[34] in short, laying down for the Algerian case what had been the fundamentals of the Hippocratic regimen for 20 centuries.

Bertherand did not perceive that the disintegration of indigenous educational institutions had been caused by foreign invasion. He considered the beliefs and practices he described to be a jumble of superstitions and empirical devices. He was blind to the internal logic of an Arab medicine which reflected the tradition that moulded his own way of thinking. Bertherand did not comment on the resistance offered to Western practices by the *tabib* (to be distinguished from the *hakim,* as being more oriented towards theoretical knowledge).

But he did mention the high esteem in which the Arabs held science and medical knowledge.[35]

At the same time, the Tunisian minister Khayr-ad-Din acknowledged Western superiority in science in a book dedicated to the reformation of Muslim states and ascribed this pre-eminence to the existence of democratic institutions.[36] In a tribute to the high status of medical knowledge in Arab culture,[37] Khayr-ad-Din welcomed the advent of 'physicians taking care of the nation's affairs', a bold metaphor that anticipated the coming to political power of physicians in the following generation.

The close linkage between the learned tradition of Arab medicine and Western science will make it difficult in the post-independence era to reinvent a national brand of medicine, as has been the case in India and China.[38] The early emergence of a secular trend in Arab medicine will also make it difficult to consider it as underlying religious revivalism. The Hippocratic tradition referred to a humoralism that had banned the supernatural. Arab medicine was never part of the Islamic sciences, not merely because its representatives belonged to the three 'Families of the Book',[39] although it developed in a social and political context framed by the *shari'a* and the needs of the Muslim faith. Only the tradition of Prophetic medicine, *Tibb an Nabi,* readily accommodates the claim to a distinct kind of non-Western science, opposed to materialistic, atheistic Western science, more concerned with the well-being of bodies than with the state of souls. In the same spirit, it is difficult to assess the degree of resistance to Western medicine, and to differentiate between the reactions of the learned and the social leaders, and the numerous *tollab* who performed cures in villages and cities.

Tropical Medicine and Mutual Rejection

Around 1890 the medical corporation began its irresistible march to power. In Algeria the dreams of an Arab kingdom once toyed with by Emperor Napoleon III had long since vanished.[40] Settlers were aware of their growing strength and of their rights on the land. The Muslim population remained segregated from the conquerors and only a minority was admitted to European schools. The medical school in Algiers, founded the first time in 1836 and re-opened in 1852, illustrated the intellectual vitality of the colony.[41] Doctors had officially made an alliance with science, solemnized by the building of the Pasteur Institute in Paris in 1888.[42] The Pastorian discoveries were immediately reported and commented on in the medical gazettes and the journals of the learned societies of Algeria. The Pasteur Institute in

Algiers was founded in 1894 by two local professors, Trolard and Soulié, to apply Pasteur's discoveries to Algeria.[43] They adhered to the Pastorian programme that typically associated the glorious past (the production of the Jennerian vaccine), the rather meagre present (the preventive treatment of anthrax and rabies),[44] and the grand future (the investigation into potential vaccines against all diseases). This local initiative bore testimony to the adoption of the new scientific agenda by the medical élite.

Doctors were no longer bringing up the rear of the army: they were to the front and even in the vanguard. The distinction between military and civilian doctors was deliberately blurred. The medical dispensary, oriented towards curing the natives, was an important part of colonial strategy, as is suggested by Marshall Lyautey's famous statement to his superiors when he was in Madagascar: 'Send me four doctors, I will send you back four battalions!'[45] Doctors could attract the sympathy of the sick and recruit supporters for French colonization, and thanks to their practice in the homes of Algerians, they constituted a unique source of information, although quite a few doctors in Morocco paid with their lives for this ambiguous role.[46]

Consistent with the scientific agenda of the Third Republic, the Pastorian school offered a programme for investigating local diseases. Pastorians attempted to put their finger on the intersection of causal mechanisms in order to interrupt disease transmission in an easy way that saved money and lives: they looked for the 'fissure', the 'crack' in Emile Duclaux's terms,[47] which made the reservoir of drinking water communicate with the sewers (to cite one instance among many). Pasteur had celebrated the merits of simple causality versus the complex factors invoked by hygienists of the former generation: 'never will poverty be able to create disease'. The mosquito theory, under way in the 1880s,[48] did not contradict the scheme of bacterial infectivity. It pointed to a supplementary weak point in the transmission pattern and suggested complementary strategies.

The small group of Pasteur's disciples gathered around the master, and enboldened by the early successes of anthrax and rabies, firmly believed in the dawn of a new medical era,[49] long before the programme had achieved any demonstrable result in demographic terms.[50] They believed that the new scientific paradigm of medicine was universally applicable. Epidemiological knowledge required identification of the initial foci of infection in order to capture the nascent pestilence. Microbiologists had to explore the sources of diseases, in the same way that geographers had to trace the sources of the Nile or the Zambesi. Pasteur was represented as the pioneer of missionary science. He himself had ventured down to Saint-Nazaire, a port on the Atlantic coast, in order to observe an epidemic of yellow fever, but firmly declined all invitations from the Emperor of Brazil to come and study the terrible disease *in situ.*[51] Tropical countries, where some diseases were rampant,[52] figured promisingly on his agenda. The scientific hurricane was moving toward the tropics and reached the Maghreb on the way. Tropical medicine demonstrated the excellence of European medicine and created satellite centres of research[53] which then to some extent, vied with the metropolitan institutions themselves.[54]

The new scientific missionaries, travelling with microscopes rather than Gospels in their pockets, did not necessarily see the link between scientific and political imperialism.[55] They did not perceive the extent to which coercive measures might be applied more easily among populations in the colonies than in the metropolis and in countries under French control rather than in foreign territories. In other words, they ignored the fact that the paradigm shift bore not only a scientific content but also a political aspect and that management by the state of medical affairs now signified modernity.[56]

Pasteur and his successors, Emile Duclaux and Emile Roux, corresponded with ministers, ambassadors and sovereigns. When they were solicited by local authorities to send experts into foreign lands, they did so eagerly, with the firm conviction that they would demonstrate their scientific superiority and eclipse their competitors. Emile Roux aspired to win for his disciples the title of 'the people's scientific schoolteachers'. The Pastorians neglected the lessons of some failures that might have alerted them to the 'political connection' of the new medicine. However, several of these failures clearly indicated that if the connection was omitted the Pastorian programme could not function. In Australia, the mission of Adrien Loir, Pasteur's nephew, was one of these failures.[57] The Pouilly-le-Fort demonstration of anthrax vaccination on a small farm was hard to reproduce on a continental scale, with thousands of cattle scattered over hundreds of square miles, despite repeated angry telegrams from Loir's formidable uncle. In a similar way, in another non-European territory, the Ottoman Empire, the mission initiated by the Pastorian hygienist André Chantemesse, sent to Constantinople in 1893 and followed by the establishment of a Pasteur-like institute, had equally dubious results.[58] The Sultan had perfectly grasped that the Pastorian doctrine was a sign of modernity. But soon after Maurice Nicolle had been appointed as head of the Ottoman Institute of Bacteriology, the local administration opposed the hygienic measures recommended by the bacteriologists. Maurice Nicolle resigned in 1899 and returned to Paris. The case of Mexico also helps to document the link between political will and the adoption of the scientific agenda. The Pastorian centre for rabies treatment was transferred to Mexico in 1888 under the control of Dr Eduardo Liceaga, Porfirio Diaz's own physician and head of the Public Health Committee. Once again received as a symbol of the new science, the imported institution did not evolve into a fully-fledged institution for medical research. Only the prestige elements of the Pastorian programme were retained, at the expense of the global programme aimed at by Pastorian ideology.

The triumph of the new scientific medicine required the fulfilment of certain political conditions and the scientists' collaboration with political and administrative structures. The conditions for fulfilling this agenda were paramount in colonial countries where political considerations did not restrict the infringement of individual rights to hygienists. Sergent remarks, for example, that it has been impossible to administer quinine to Europeans as an effective prophylaxis,[59] and that the target of sanitary campaigns should be the natives. The distinctive mark of these campaigns was the use, whether manifest or not, of coercion. The perfect example of this were the campaigns to enforce smallpox vaccination and their counterpart, the repression of the inoculation still practised in the Algerian countryside.[60] Yet this was also true for most measures linked to public health, such as the control of migration and the frequent interdiction of pilgrimages to Mecca under the pretext of cholera or plague epidemics in the Middle East.[61] In the realm of health, the 'angles morts', according to Lyautey,[62] should not exist, a view suggestive of a Foucaultian Panopticon.[63] Meanwhile, the idea of preventive medicine imposed by the state was only slowly making its way in the metropolis. Forty years of parliamentary debate resulted in the 1902 law on compulsory smallpox vaccination: in many ways this legislation had already been anticipated in Algeria and Indochina. But these social and political factors were never officially recognized as key factors in the success of Pastorian innovations.

In contrast to the former generation, Pasteur adopted a more aggressive attitude in matters of public health and followed an activist agenda characterized as 'transformist' by his devotees. A famous member of the French Society of Anthropology said in a public conference that 'Pasteur was Lamarck plus Darwin'.[64] In his programme of virus attenuation, Pasteur manipulated germs: he successively adapted them to different media, then selected them.[65] Transformism meant activism, contrasted by the colonial party to the alleged fatalism of the Muslim population,[66] who were held responsible for the bad quality of their milieu (the concept of 'guilty social space').[67] Another aspect of this activist doctrine was the interception of disease transmission in the field. This attitude was the opposite of *laissez-faire,* but the study of the epidemiological cycle was planned to detect one or several weak links in order to interrupt transmission. Such a programme, has recently been revived, just as the issue of 'globalism' has recently been re-opened in the debate on a preventive strategy for Aids.[68]

The reception of Laveran's parasite, after his description of it in 1880 at Constantine,[69] was not immediately enthusiastic in the group surrounding Pasteur. There was an abyss between the simple morphology of cocci and bacilli and the elusive polymorphic parasite observed by Laveran on the surface, not inside, red blood cells.[70] These doubts were to disappear from the official version of the discovery. For Laveran's jubilee in 1915, Emile Roux polished the final version of the myth by attributing the official acknowledgement of the discovery to Pasteur himself. 'Something alive, immediately recognizable as a living pathogen, was moving restlessly under the microscope.'[71]

The Pastorians wiped their memories clean and edited the past. They rejected the medicine of warm climates as well as ancient notions of hygiene.[72] They pushed it back into what the American physician William Osler called 'Egyptian darkness'. Only recently have the difficulties encountered by campaigns for the eradication of parasitic diseases, by re-imposing an environmental mode of thought, led geographers and epidemiologists to revive the work of the pioneers of medical geography.[73]

Malaria, the Crux of Tropical Medicine

Once the role of the plasmodium was admitted, it did not take long for Emile Roux to experiment with the mosquito theory in the field, following Koch in India and Grassi in Italy. In 1902, at the request of Governor Jonnart himself, Roux dispatched to Algiers the brothers Edmond and Etienne Sergent, both from the Medical School of Algiers but trained at the Pasteur Institute. It was not their first mission. They chose as an observatory, a place where malaria transmission was intense, the railway station at Alma in the Mitidja plain, an attractive place for settlers because of its proximity to Algiers and its reputed fertility. Farmers settled close to the railway embankments where they would bring their stock for market. The permanent gathering of mixed sedentary and nomadic crowds around railway stations multiplied the number of malaria cases in the population. Ponds linked to daily human activities and irrigation channels provided many breeding sites for larvae. The 'railway phenomenon' was also identified in malaria surveys in India,[74] and suggested the ambivalent benefits of technological innovation.

The Sergents' method of 'anti-paludism' was eclectic. It combined Koch's method – quinine treatment[75] – with mosquito screens on doors and windows, and drainage as recommended by the Italians. It called for the removal of weeds from canal banks and the spreading of oil on the surface of stagnant water in order to destroy the larvae, the stage of the insect's life most vulnerable to anti-mosquito measures. A battle-dress reminiscent of medieval anti-plague garments was designed for employees on duty during the night, but rapidly proved unpopular.

The alleged results of the measures conducted on the scale of the small station were so good that the Sergent brothers were appointed to the sanitary surveillance of the entire railway network. The 'railway campaign' was described as the equivalent of the famous Pasteur demonstration of anthrax vaccination at the farm of Pouilly-le-Fort in Beauce.[76] Pastorian science received the support of the same social group who had patronized Pasteur's early endeavours in the field of public health. Thus there was no surprise when, in 1907, the Pastorian group evicted the former staff of the Algiers Institute and put Calmette at its head.[77] Edmond Sergent officially succeeded Calmette in 1910. The Sergent Brothers chose 'anti-paludism' as their touchstone and the emblem of the new Pastorian medicine. Field studies and interventions came side-by-side with the production of sera and vaccines, in the typical combination of basic research and applied science that was becoming the stamp of Pastorian medicine.

In 1911, Emile Roux, who seldom travelled, paid a visit to Algiers for the official inauguration of the Institute at its new premises. Edmond Sergent tells the story in his book *History of an Algerian Marsh*, published in 1947, a good example of the Pastorian quest for a founding myth:[78]

> On a golden evening in May 1911, the car drove toward Algiers... We came back with our master Dr Roux from Montebello village, where we had shown him our 'field of anti-paludic experimentation'; for eight years we had tested the new methods inspired by Ross and Laveran's discoveries. Suddenly, Dr Roux whose piercing eyes scrutinize everything, exclaims: 'What does this abandoned farm mean?' On the road side, an isolated house stands, barricaded with closed shutters. Solitude and silence. The desertion epitomizes the malaria nightmare in Algeria.

After thinking for a while, Emile Roux dictated his orders:

> Here is what you must do. Look for a place which is not inhabited because of malaria. You will position healthy farmers[79] there, you will protect them and sanitize the soil using all the methods which you have already experimented with. You will demonstrate that rational methods will lead to the conquest of malaria. Let it be shown beyond any doubt (Que la preuve éclate!), that an innocuous, rapid and definitive sanitization is possible.

The anecdote is a typical masterpiece of Pastorian hagiography. The anecdote sets the stage for a further demonstration which in turn culminates in public acceptance. Popularization was an integral part of Pastorian science and amplified its scope and action. The systematic search for 'special effects' anticipates the modern manipulation of the masses.

In his passionate account, Emile Roux combines methods of combating malaria already familiar on the scene of the Ouled Mendil marshes. The choice of the theatre is by no means fortuitous: the isolated farm is in the centre of a fertile piece of land, all very promising. The scientific demonstration is necessary for the programme of 'integral improvement' of soils in close proximity to the Algerian capital.[80] Two-thirds of the Mitidja plain are allegedly left uncultivated while the demand for land is growing.[81]

In subsequent reports Sergent detailed his epidemiological research.[82] The Algerians are the target of mass investigation. The campaigns are to determine the epidemiological indexes that are appropriate markers for the assessment of malaria endemicity. The splenic index, for instance, requires only the palpation of the enlarged spleen in the left hypochondrium. Sergent remarks that clinical examination is easy with naked-bellied young children or even with adults: men can be examined on the street after untying their belts. We are very far from the cosy atmosphere of a medical office. Sergent's vision followed a new scientific pattern. The natives were segregated in epidemiological discourse as well as in method of treatment in the field. According to a transparent metaphor,[83] the parasite was the germ, the European was the soil, and the natives were the reservoir.[84] Being germ carriers, they came to be identified with the germs themselves: 'The contaminated subjects play the same role as the "pieds de cuve" in fermentation.'[85] The indigenous population posed the main epidemic threat to the settlers. In pictures the proximity of the infected *gourbi* to the opulent farm illustrated the dangers of being so close.[86] In the Algerian landscape, as depicted by Sergent, the natives were part of the natural environment, which was the antithesis of civilization. This environment was to be radically transformed by the settlers' activity and Algeria would return to Roman prosperity.[87] Systematic quininization of the virus reservoir [meaning the indigenous people] develops their working potential and productivity and results in the growing prosperity of the natives, torn from their primitive barbary by French science and energy.[88]

No attention was paid to the anthropological and social issues raised by the new strategies. The earlier medicine of warm climates, more sensitive to these issues and envisioning a mixed society, was forgotten. The archetype of the new epidemiology was one of a natural environment where exhaustive description was possible, given the limited number of significant parameters:

> Une oasis isolée comme une ile dans la mer offre un milieu idéal pour l'étude du mode de transmission d'une maladie épidémique qui s'y propage en vase clos. Flore, faune, populations sont connues, cataloguées. Aucun élément étranger ne peut pénétrer à l'insu du médecin dans ce milieu fermé et isolé.[89]

The conquistador epistemology of the Sergent brothers clearly displayed a blind spot: the doctor's position which determined the co-ordinates of the whole field. No one could penetrate unseen the oasis, the island in the desert, no one, that is, except the doctor, invisible in his own eyes, embodying the recent perturbations of germ traffic.

The Sergents envisioned medical activism as an entirely positive enterprise. WHO officers echoed their optimistic line when in the 1960s they adopted the agenda of disease eradication. However, not all Pastorians were so blind to the complexities of epidemiological analysis. Some of the colonial doctors had a more sober view and between the lines one can perceive two disturbing factors in the picture: on one hand, the autonomous dynamics of 'epidemic genius'; on the other hand, the gross mutations of pathology triggered by the political, social and economic changes that occurred in Africa and Asia,[90] in less than a century.[91] Dr Eugène Jamot's campaign against sleeping sickness in Equatorial Africa between the two world wars,[92] has been celebrated as another great success for 'Pastorian methods', combining mass detection and treatment. Historians today emphasize how the outburst of epidemics was linked to a radical change in the scale of human trade and migration, with the intensive labour and military conscription imposed by colonialism. Ironically, colonialism has contributed to combating a fire which it had in great part kindled. This is an historical paradox which the Pastorian Charles Nicolle has not ignored for Tunis. Demographic data, today being re-investigated, pointed to population stagnation.[93] Being given the high fecundity rate, this stagnation[94] resulted from the combination of persisting 'medieval' pestilences (such as plague) with the explosion of typhus and tuberculosis as a consequence of urbanization and over-crowding[95] – a clear illustration of what has been named the 'epidemiological transition'.[96]

'Detropicalizing' Algeria

Tropical medicine in Pastorian times was invoked in two important scientific contexts. On the one hand, the laboratory model of microbiology (virus attenuation, experimental studies on animals), and the field studies of parasitology on the other hand, dominated by vector-transmitted diseases and the notion of natural cycles, a suggestion offered for dissecting the complexities of environmental interactions. The Pastorian agenda and its triumphalist ethos favoured microbiology over parasitology, the action over the germ-carrier, the human reservoir over the global perspective.

In their successes, the Pastorians clearly benefited from the political context. But the scientific paradigm of tropical medicine was unstable, because of the unsolved opposition between a reductionist view and a more holistic approach to disease. The eclipse of the discipline, in the post-colonial era, as soon as political conditions were no longer favourable to a certain scientific style, is witness to this instability linked to the hybrid nature of the underlying paradigm and to dependence on the historical context. Contemporary studies may lead to a re-appraisal of the picture of malaria management in North Africa before and during the conquest, which differs from the epic told by the Sergents. The metaphor of tropical medicine has blurred the vision of epidemiological realities. The Mitidja experiment, the Algerian counterpart of Pouilly-le-Fort, allegedly provided the proof of the superiority of French science. But the story is not complete unless it says more about the disappointments of the small settlers' craving for land, the ambitions of the landowners residing in Algiers and the migration of Arabs to find a refuge on the inhospitable slopes of the surrounding mountains.

Lastly, the modern understanding of the epidemiological complexities of malaria transmission also leads to a more sober appreciation of the Pastorian campaigns that resulted in its present eradication and raises many questions. The plasmodium described by Laveran was undoubtedly *Plasmodium falciparum,* which explains the high fatality rate of malarial fevers in the middle of the century. At the same time, this northern extension of the plasmodium of tropical climates may have been very unstable and its biotope not well established. Another hypothesis is that mortality was caused by a once more virulent *Plasmodium vivax*. Today, malaria has been practically eradicated from North Africa, except in a few oases, and only *P. vivax* is found. After all, Algeria was not quite tropical in the hard sense of the word, and the Pastorians had rather an easy time of it.

Notes

1. M. Worboys, 'The emergence of tropical medicine: A study in the establishment of a scientific specialty', in G. Lemaine, R. MacLeod and M. Mulkay (eds), *Perspectives on the Emergence of Scientific Disciplines,* (The Hague: Mouton, 1976), 75–98.
2. A. M. Moulin, 'Bacteriological research and medical practice in and outside the Pasteurian school', in Ann LaBerge and M. Feingold (eds), *French Medical Culture in the Nineteenth Century,* 327–49.
3. M. Bruneau and D. Dory, *Les enjeux de la tropicalité,* (Paris: Masson, 1989).
4. C. Lévi-Strauss, *Tristes tropiques,* (Paris: Plon, 1955).
5. P. Gourou, *Terres de bonne espérance: Le monde tropical,* (Paris: Plon, 1972).
6. For the general background of French colonial history, see J. Meyer *et al.* (eds), *Histoire de la France coloniale des origines à 1914,* (Paris: 1991).
7. P. D. Curtin, 'The White Man's Grave: Image and reality: 1780–1850', *Journal of British Studies,* 1 (1961), 94–110.
8. J. Theodoridès, 'La contribution française à la parasitologie médicale et à la pathologie exotique de 1900 à 1950, *Histoire des sciences médicales,* 3 (1993), 223–31.
9. See correspondence between Félix Mesnil and Charles Nicolle, 1904–36, Archives départementales de Seine Maritime, Rouen, Fonds Nicolle.
10. J. Theodoridès, 'La contribution de Félix Mesnil (1868–1938) à l'étude des Sporozoaires, *Histoire et Nature,* 30 (1993), 43–53.
11. J. Léonard, *La médecine entre les savoirs et les pouvoirs,* (Paris: 1981); C. Salomon-Bayet, *Pasteur et la révolution pastorienne,* (Paris: 1986); C. Rosenberg and M. Vogel (eds), *The Therapeutic Revolution: Essays in the Social History of American Medicine,* (Philadelphia: University of Pennsylvania Press, 1979).
12. L. Raynaud, Soulié et Picard, *Hygiène et pathologie nord-africaine 1830–1930,* (Paris: Masson, 1931), Vol I.
13. He was said to carry out the amputation of an upper limb in two minutes, and similarly for a lower limb.
14. L. Raynaud, *op. cit.* (note 12), Vol. 1, 202.
15. Yvonne Turin evokes 'la frange insignifiante d'une action militaire

écrasante', *Affrontements culturels dans l'Algérie coloniale: Ecoles, médecine, religion, 1830–1880* (Paris: Maspéro, 1971), 80.

16. A. M. Moulin, 'L'adversaire le plus redoutable des coloniaux : Le paludisme', G. Balandier and M. Ferro (eds), *Le Temps des Colonies,* (Paris: Seuil, 1984), 62–6.
17. J. N. Périer, 'De l'acclimatement en Algérie', *Annales d'Hygiène publique et de médecine légale,* 33 (1845), 305.
18. M.-F. Roport, 'Aux sources de la géographie de la santé: Les topographies médicales en France aux XVIIIe et XIXe siècles', *Cahiers Géos,* 21 (1991) 7–14. 820 topographies were published between 1756 and 1895, with peaks around 1825 and 1850; among these 69 alone were on Algeria alone. J.-C. Boudin coined the term 'géographie médicale' in 1843. Around 1880, the shift to a global scale is obvious in A. Bordier's *Géographie médicale* (Paris: Reinwald, 1884) and the global work of A. Hirsch, *Handbuch der Historisch-Geographischen Pathologie,* (Berlin: 1st edn, 1860, 2nd edn, 1881).
19. J.-N. Périer, *De l'hygiène en Algérie,* (Paris: 1847), 2 vols.
20. Michael Osborne has emphasized the resurrrection of the Hippocratic mode of questioning when doctors were faced with an unfamiliar situation; see his essay in this volume.
21. J.-P. Peter (ed.), *Médecine, climats et épidémies à la fin du XVIIIe siècle,* (Paris: Mouton, 1972).
22. Périer, *op. cit.* (note 17), 304.
23. E. Sergent, *Notice sur l'institut Pasteur d'Algérie,* (Algiers: Carbonel, 1934), 344–56 .
24. Cf. Sergent's statement in 1928: 'Le climat propice au blanc exclut le noir et inversement le climat propice au noir exclut le blanc.' 'Rapport sur le fonctionnement de l'institut Pasteur d'Algérie en 1927', *Archives de l'institut Pasteur d'Algérie,* 6 (1928), 61.
25. 'Les nations ne s'acclimatent et ne prennent racine en des contrées lointaines qu'avec le concours des modifications profondes qui résultent du croisement avec les indigènes', Périer, *op. cit.* (note 17), 305. For analogous statements in Indonesia, see A. L. Stoler, 'Rethinking colonial categories: European communities and the boundaries of rule', *Comparative Studies in Society and History,* 31 (1989), 134–61. This discourse suddenly stops along with the policy of importing whole families instead of finding local partners for male settlers. On both sides, the opposition to intermating was evident.
26. The advice for soldiers lists abstention from rich food, drinking alcohol in moderation, the use of wine with water, and restraint in sexual liaisons.
27. For the effectiveness of these measures, see P. D. Curtin, *Death by Migration: Europe's Encounter with the Tropical World in the Nineteenth Century,* (Cambridge: Cambridge University Press, 1989).
28. 'On contagion according to *hadiths*', B. Dinguizli, 'La variole en

Tunisie', medical doctorate thesis, Bordeaux: 1896–97; M. Dols, *The Black Death in the Middle East,* (Princeton: Princeton University Press, 1977), 109–21; L. Conrad, 'Epidemic disease in formal and popular thought in early Islamic society', in T. Ranger and P. Slack (eds), *Epidemics and Ideas,* (Cambridge: Cambridge University Press, 1992), 77–99.

29. L. Leclerc, *Histoire de la médecine arabe,* (Paris: 1876, Rabat: 1980).
30. The medical gazettes contain numerous examples of this scholarly interest. Each issue of the *Gazette médicale d'Algérie* disserts at length on pharmacopoeia, trephining, diagnosis and treatment of skin diseases among the Arabs, etc.
31. On this divergence in the Egyptian context, A. M. Moulin, 'Révolutions médicales et politiques en Egypte (1865–1917)', *Revue de l'Occident musulman et de la Méditerranée,* 2 (1989), 99–110 ; and more generally, 'La profession médicale dans les pays arabes: Vues historiques à long et à court terme: Médecins et protection sociale dans le monde arabe', in S. Chiffoleau and B. Curmi (eds), *Cahiers du CERMOC,* 5 (1993), 223–46.
32. E. L. Bertherand, *Médecine et hygiène des Arabes,* (Paris: 1855).
33. N. Gallagher, *Medicine and Power in Tunisia, 1780–1900.* (Cambridge: Cambridge University Press, 1983).
34. To avoid excessive sweating and discourage sensitivity to the reigning miasmatic atmosphere.
35. For example, the famous proverb, quoted from the *hadith*: 'study science from the cradle to the grave', and also 'go and search for science so far as China'. On Abd el Kader's library, see S. Zakri, 'Abd el Kader sur le chemin de Damas', *Qantara,* 9 (1993), 58–61.
36. 'Est-il possible que ceux qui sont destinés à être les médecins de la nation ignorent la nature du mal?', Khayr-ed-Din, *Essai sur les réformes nécessaires aux états musulmans (1867–1868),* (Paris: Edisud, 1987), 84.
37. Of course with the reservation that the superiority of Muslim countries lay in their religious faith.
38. A. M. Moulin, 'La profession médicale arabe' (note 31); B. Good and M.-J. del Vecchio-Good, 'The comparative study of Greco-Islamic medicine: The integration of medical knowledge into local symbolic contexts', C. Leslie and A. Young (eds), *Asian Paths to Medical Knowledge*, (Berkeley: University of California Press, 1992), 257–71.
39. Jews, Christians and Muslims.
40. Paul Cambon's 'enlightened projects', between 1895 and 1900, were rejected, see C. R. Ageron, *Les Algériens musulmans et la France,* (Paris: Presses universitaires de France, 1968), Vol. I, 518–27. Also H. Laurens, *Le royaume imposssible: La France et la genèse du monde arabe,* (Paris: A. Colin, 1990).
41. L. Moreau, 'L'oeuvre scientifique de l'école de médecine d'Alger', *Revue africaine,* 43 (1905), 458–62.
42. On the social rise of medical profession, see J. Léonard, C Salomon-

Bayet and J.-P. Goubert (eds), *La médicalisation de la société française, 1770–1830,* (Ontario: Historical Reflections Press, 1982) ; J. Ellis, *The Physician-Legislators of France: Medicine and Politics in the early Third Republic,* (Cambridge: Cambridge University Press, 1991); on the permanent fighting against 'quacks', M. Ramsey, *Professional and Popular Medicine in France, 1770–1830,* (Cambridge: Cambridge University Press, 1988).

43. A. M. Moulin, 'Les instituts Pasteur de la Méditerranée arabe: Une religion scientifique en pays d'islam', in E. Longuenesse (ed.), *Santé et société dans le monde arabe,* (Paris: L'Harmattan, forthcoming).
44. I have tried elsehere to prove that Pasteur incorporated the Jennerian past into the fabric of his own work: A. M. Moulin, 'La métaphore vaccine: De l'inoculation à la vaccinologie', *History and Philosophy of Life Sciences,*14 (1993), 271–97.
45. On Lyautey and medicine, see D. Rivet, 'Hygiènisme colonial et médicalisation de la société marocaine au temps du protectorat français, 1912–1956', in Longuenesse, *op. cit.* (note 43).
46. J. Paul, 'Medicine and imperialism in Morocco', MERIP, 60 (1977) 3.
47. E. Duclaux, *L'Hygiène sociale,* (Paris: Aldan, 1902).
48. F. Delaporte, *Histoire de la fièvre jaune,* (Paris: Rayot, 1991).
49. Moulin, *op. cit.* (note 2).
50. On the demographic effects of pre-Pastorian hygienic measures, notably in colonial armies, see Curtin, *op. cit.* (note 27). On demography in the Arab world, see Y. Courbage and P. Fargues, *Chrétiens et Juifs dans l'Islam arabe et turc,* (Paris: Fayard, 1992).
51. L. Pasteur, Letters to Emperor Don Pedro, 1891, Correspondence, Bibliothèque nationale.
52. Arriving at Tangiers in 1911, Remlinger complained that the climate in Morocco did not greatly differ from that in Europe and left little chance of making distinguished discoveries in microbiology.
53. A. M. Moulin, 'Charles Nicolle, médecin tunisien', *Archives de l'institut Pasteur de Tunis,* forthcoming.
54. Tensions would appear between the Pasteur Institute in Paris, trying to retain a monopoly of basic research and the self-assertive overseas branches, A. M. Moulin, 'Patriarchal science: The research work of the overseas Pasteur Institute', in P. Petitjean, C. Jami and A. M. Moulin (eds), *Science and Empires,* (Boston: Kluwer, 1992), 307–22.
55. On the alliance of Western medicine with the political, military and economic needs of imperialism in the years 1870–1914, see D. Arnold (ed.), *Imperial Medicine and Indigenous Societies* (Manchester: Manchester University Press, 1988).
56. See P. Boomgaard's remarks on the importance of state medicine in Indonesia in this volume.
57. J. Chaussivert, *'L'institut Pasteur d'Australie',* in M. Morange (ed.), *L'institut Pasteur. Contributions à son histoire,* (Paris: La Découverte, 1991), 242–53.

58. A. M. Moulin, 'L'hygiène dans la ville: La médecine pastorienne à l'heure ottomane', in F. Georgeon et P. Dumont (eds), in *Les villes ottomanes à la fin de l'empire,* (Paris: L'Harmattan, 1992), 145–67 .
59. 'La défense mécanique et la quininisation préventive d'une population européenne ne sont pas mesures dont l'Etat doive assumer l'application. L'Etat ne peut ni les imposer ni en contrôler l'importance.' E. Sergent, 'Vingt-cinq années d'études du paludisme', *Archives de l'institut Pasteur d'Algérie,* 6 (1928),142.
60. On smallpox vaccination in Algeria and the suppression of inoculation, see P. Trolard, 'Des mesures à prendre pour propager la vaccine en territoire indigène', (Algiers: Giralt, 1900).
61. Raynaud, *op. cit.* (note 12).
62. Maréchal Lyautey, 26 June,1926, *Paroles d'action,* (Paris: A. Colin,1927), 444, quoted by Rivet, *op. cit.* (note 45).
63. M. Foucault, *Surveiller et punir* (Paris: Gallimard, 1968).
64. A Bordier, 'Les microbes et le transformisme', *Bulletin de la Société d'Anthropologie de Paris',11* (1988) 743.
65. A. M. Moulin, *Le dernier langage de la médecine: Histoire de l'immunologie de Pasteur au SIDA,* (Paris: Presses universitaires de France, 1991), Ch 1.
66. G. Hardy, Géographie et colonisation, (Paris: Gallimard, 1933), 18: 'C'est le propre des oeuvres de colonisation de fournir à l'initiative humaine un champ fort étendu.'
67. J. P. Hervouët and C. Laveissière, 'Les grandes endémies, l'espace social coupable', *Politique africaine,* 28 (1987), 21–32.
68. J. Mann, D. Tarantola and T. W. Netter (eds), *AIDS in the World. The Global AIDS Policy Coalition,* (Cambridge, Mass.: Harvard University Press, 1992).
69. E. Sergent, 'La découverte de Laveran', *Collection du centenaire de l'Algérie,* On Laveran see M. Phisalix, *Alphonse Laveran, sa vie, son oeuvre,* (Paris: Masson, 1923).
70. A. Laveran, 'Protozoa as the causes of diseases', Nobel Lectures, *Physiology and Medicine,* (Amsterdam: Elsevier, 1907), 264–71.
71. E. Roux, 'Discours à l'occasion du jubilé de M Le professeur Laveran', *Annales de l'institut Pasteur,* 29 (1915), 405.
72. A. LaBerge, *Mission and Method: The Early Nineteenth Century French Public Health Movement,* (Cambridge: Cambridge University Press, 1992).
73. H. Picheral and G. Salem, 'De la géographie médicale à la géographie de la santé', *Cahiers Geos,* 22 (1992).
74. The epidemiological importance of railway stations in India had been emphasized even before 1880: see I. Klein, 'Death in India 1871–1921', *Journal of Asian Studies,* 32 (1973), 639–59.
75. Diverging from Koch, who prescribed a gramme of quinine every two weeks, they administered quinine daily at low doses and did not check the blood slides. Their treatment was both preventive and curative.

76. On the role of 'le théâtre de la preuve, see B. Latour, *The Pasteurization of France,* (Cambridge, Mass.: Harvard University Press, 1988).
77. P. Trolard, *L'institut Pasteur d'Alger: Sa fondation: Sa réorganisation: Mon expulsion,* (Algiers: Imprimerie orientale, 1910).
78. E. Sergent and E. Sergent, *Histoire d'un marais algérien,* (Algiers: Institut Pasteur d'Algérie, 1847), 7–9.
79. A euphemism for European settlers.
80. On the financial and social aspects of this capitalist venture, see G. Morin, 'Le chef d'oeuvre de la France, la Mitidja', *Le Temps des colonies,* 84–92.
81. I. Hamet, *Les musulmans français du Nord de l'Afrique,* (Paris: A. Colin, 1906), 244–5.
82. E. Sergent, *Travaux scientifiques sur l'institut Pasteur d'Algérie de 1900 à 1962,* (Paris: Presses universitaires de France, 1963).
83. On the ambivalent dangers of the parasite/parasite-carrier in the period of post-war eradication, see P. Weindling, 'Medicine and Holocaust: The case of typhus', I. Löwy (ed.), *Medicine and Change: Historical and Sociological Studies of Medical Innovation,* (Montrouge: John Libbey, 1993), 447–64.
84. Sergent, *op. cit.* (note 23).
85. Sergent, *op. cit.* (note 59), 121.
86. *Ibid.*, where the picture on page 235 corroborates the text on page 234.
87. The South African myth for North Africa, as observed by Fanny Colonna, 15 March, 1993.
88. Sergent, *op. cit.* (note 59), 234.
89. *Ibid.*, 122
90. G. W. Hartwig and K. D. Patterson (eds), *Disease in African History: An Introductory Survey and Case Studies,* (Durham: Duke University Press, 1978).
91. J.-P. Dozon, 'Quand les Pastoriens traquaient la maladie du sommeil', *Sciences sociales et santé,* 3 (1985), 27–56.
92. M. Bebey Eyidi, Le vainqueur de la maladie du sommeil, le docteur Eugène Jamot (1879–1937), (Paris: 1950); Lapeyssonnie, *Médecine coloniale. Mythes et réalités* (Paris: Seghers, 1988).
93. A. Loir, 'Statistique de la population de Tunis', *Revue Tunisienne,* 5 (1898), 348–53.
94. *La démographie historique en Tunisie et dans le monde arabe,* Actes du colloque des 15 et 16 Novembre, (Tunis: Cérès Productions, 1993).
95. See, for example, D. Rivet, 'La recrudescence des épidémies au Maroc durant la deuxième guerre mondiale: Essai de mesure et d'interprétation, *Hespéris,* 30 (1992), 93–109.
96. A. R. Omran, 'The epidemiological transition', *Millbank Memorial Bank Quarterly,* 49 (1971), 509–38.

9

Germs, Malaria and the Invention of Mansonian Tropical Medicine: From 'Diseases in the Tropics' to 'Tropical Diseases'

Michael Worboys

The transfer of the germ theory of disease to the problem of disease in the tropics was once regarded as a sufficient condition for the emergence of Mansonian tropical medicine.[1] More recently, historians have given greater prominence to social and political considerations, but the cognitive framework provided by germ theory is still given a pivotal role.[2] So what was this all-important theory? At its simplest it was the proposition that microscopic organisms were the causes of specific infectious and contagious diseases. Historically it has been associated with the development of bacteriology, with Pasteur, Koch and Lister celebrated as the triumvirate that brought germs from theory to fact.[3] Manson certainly saw his work as part of this larger programme of converting zymotic afflictions to germ diseases.[4] Yet Mansonian tropical medicine was not built upon the foundations of bacteriology; instead it became synonymous with non-bacterial diseases caused by unicellular and multicellular organisms (protozoa and helminths) transmitted by insects and other vectors – what are now known as parasitic diseases.

The extent to which germs were seen as parasitic and parasites as the germs of disease is an interesting question, and not just for historians. The separation of bacteriology and virology from parasitology has meant that both specialisms have not learned as much from each other as they could.[5] John Farley has suggested that for most of the nineteenth century 'the world of parasites was quite distinct from the world of infectious diseases' and that the opportunities to build a unified parasitic germ theory of disease were not taken.[6] This claim seems to me to underestimate the variability and malleability of germ theories in the last quarter of the nineteenth century, and not to give sufficient weight to those cases where the nature of any germ was uncertain for many years, as was the case with malaria. My contention is that the scientific legitimation of Manson's definition of tropical medicine, rather than confirming an agreed distinction between parasitic and infectious diseases, actually created that division and that it only developed from the very end of the century. On top of this, I will argue that the character of Mansonian tropical medicine owed as much to its distinctive approach to disease control as to its cognitive framework.

A more general objection to the notion of the transfer of germ theory to medicine in the tropics is that there was not a single or simple germ theory. Rather there were several and competing theories about the nature, spread and action of germs. Many of these views can be seen as the products of distinct professional groups and were shaped by their interests and work.[7] With this more eclectic and socially grounded view of germ theories other things follow. First, developing germ practices, the techniques of seeing and manipulating microbes, deserve as much attention as germ theories. Also, that many existing medical and sanitary procedures, such as disinfection, isolation and vaccination, were re-defined as germ practices. Second, the nature of germs and their actions cannot be considered in isolation from ideas about the body's reactions to them. In other words, the histories of bacteriology and immunology, pathogen and body defences, 'seed' and 'soil', have to be seen as two sides of the same coin. Third, germ ideas and practices were not just a set of cognitive and technical innovations, but were important carriers of new meanings for science in medicine, and of specific, ontological conceptions of disease.[8] Fourth, all these ideas and practices were open to different interpretations and consequently, very different meanings about their implications for the nature and control of diseases were drawn. For example, Koch's identification of the tubercle bacillus as the necessary cause of tuberculosis not only led to an interest in destroying the 'seeds' of this disease and preventing their spread, it also led to questions about why these 'seeds' produced such variable results in different individuals and to attempts to modify the human soil to make it more resistant.[9] Clearly, any relation between germ ideas, practices and meanings, and Mansonian tropical medicine needs careful delineation.

This essay is in three parts and is mainly about events in Britain and the British Empire, where Mansonian tropical medicine was first institutionalized. The first section discusses how 'diseases in the tropics', notably fevers, were understood and managed in the middle decades of the nineteenth century. I suggest that while there were discourses on the special diseases of the tropics, these were increasingly set in the same terms as the dominant European medical systems, where all disease was seen as specific and yet could vary according to person, time and place. In short, doctors practised (ordinary) medicine in the tropics, not a distinct kind of (tropical) medicine. Next, I will discuss changing ideas about the nature and management of what came to be seen as the most serious 'disease in the tropics' – malarial fever. I consider the consequence of this becoming a candidate for a germ aetiology, the variety of accounts proposed, and the conditions which brought about the closure of medical opinion around a particular aetiological account – infection by a protozoan and transmission by a mosquito vector. Finally, I consider how malaria ceased to be a 'disease in the tropics' and became the paradigmatic Mansonian 'tropical disease'. Here I consider the often neglected practical arm of Mansonian tropical medicine – 'tropical hygiene' – and how its programme of disease control diverged from contemporary European public health policies.[10]

Diseases in the Tropics

In the middle decades of the nineteenth century there were two main discourses on disease in the tropics: the oldest gave advice to individual European travellers, traders and colonialists on the maintenance of individual health, while a newer literature was concerned with the health of European settlements in terms of sanitation.[11] The manuals on individual health tended to have their origins in advice on survival in one area, usually the West Indies or India, though by mid-century they were often addressing a growing market for advice on tropical zones across the world. Most claimed that the high levels of mortality and morbidity experienced in tropical regions had been and could be reduced further. A core assumption was that high and fluctuating temperatures, high humidity, and exposure to intense sunlight weakened the constitutions of Europeans who were not designed for, or adapted to, warm climates. Early nineteenth-century texts still spoke in humoral terms of the blood throwing off 'fiery and acrid elements' in the form of fever, 'prickly heat' and leg ulcers, though by mid-century this had been recast in terms of pathological anatomy and physiology, with excessive heat said to disrupt normal circulation and nutrition, or to diminish the metabolism of the internal organs, especially the stomach and liver.[12]

In such an abnormal and delicately balanced state, Europeans were seen to be vulnerable to all diseases, with a strong predisposition to fevers, particularly in areas where there was bad air (malaria).

Coping with such a situation demanded a strict regimen of clothing, diet, exercise, control of the 'passions', and the avoidance of shocks to the system.[13] Some believed that in time European constitutions would adjust and that acclimatization would allow settlement of the tropics. However, such optimism was becoming rarer after mid-century as anti-acclimatizationists, drawing increasingly upon evolutionary arguments, stressed the adaptation of different races to different environments. In these terms, Europeans might only adapt to the tropics through an infusion of native blood, or be able to survive by short posting and frequent returns to temperate climes to allow the body to regain equilibrium and strength.[14] Perhaps this growing pessimism reflected the experience, recently revealed by Curtin, that the steep fall in European mortality in the tropics seen in the first half of the century levelled out relatively from the 1850s.[15] However, mortality was only one of many factors, cultural, political and social, that shaped European perceptions of the tropics and their peoples.

After 1850, increasing attention was given to the health of European communities in the tropics in terms of sanitary conditions. In this sphere there was again a transfer of ideas and practices from Europe; indeed, sanitarians often compared the working-class districts of British industrial cities with 'darkest Africa' and 'teeming Asia'.[16] They supposed that the same factors that produced poisonous atmospheres in British cities, principally sanitary neglect, simply wrought a higher toll in more backward colonies. 'Asiatic cholera' was very important to this perspective.[17] It was a disease which, while endemic to India, had spread across the world and thrived in insanitary conditions at nearly every latitude.

The most important setting for the transfer of sanitarianism at this time was military hygiene. The Royal Commission on the Sanitary State of the Indian Army concluded in its report in 1863 that while temperature and moisture caused a certain amount of sickness, of greater significance were the 'other causes of a very active kind, connected with stations, barracks, hospitals, and the habits of the men, of the same nature as those which are known in colder climates to occasion attacks of those very diseases from which the Indian Army suffer so severely'.[18] As David Arnold has shown, it was political and logistic factors which inhibited state medicine in India, not uncertainties over the disease environment and its management.[19] Parkes' *Manual of Practical Hygiene,* published in 1864, based on both Indian and British experience, offered an exemplary sanitarian approach.[20] Parkes did not speak of India as a tropical country, but one where there was an 'immense variety of temperature' and 'range of humidity'; he pointed to the 'special hygienic conditions (apart from locality)' as the main causes of the excess of disease.[21] The final section of the *Manual,* which discussed overseas service, was written in terms of the problems of particular stations, not in terms of anything generally or uniquely tropical. When discussing the West Indies, Parkes spoke of earlier times when everything was blamed on the 'dreaded climate', whereas 'it is now fully recognised that ... the same customs will insure the same results. Apart from malaria, we hold our health and life almost at will'.[22] The 1891 revision of the *Manual,* edited by James Notter, repeated earlier observations about the minor influence of climate.

> India presents in many respects the same history as our other tropical possessions. In former times there was a large mortality among Europeans, attributed usually to the climate, instead of being put down to its proper causes, viz., a reckless mode of living amidst the most insanitary conditions.[23]

In the last quarter of the nineteenth century doctors and sanitary officials were increasingly confident about the potential of sanitary measures and the relatively minor role played by climate as such.[24]

While the discourses on individual constitutional protection and sanitary precautions can be presented as conflicting – internal/bodily versus external/environmental – most colonialists found them complementary, or had no trouble trying to stay alive with the contradictions. Both discourses agreed that the serious diseases of the tropics were analogous to those found in temperate climes and could be combated by variations on standard European approaches. Categories like those of continuous, intermittent and remittent fever worked as well in Madras as in Manchester, Bermuda as Birmingham, Lagos as London. Differences were of degree rather than kind. Mark Harrison's recent caution that colonial medical practitioners often felt that 'the degree was sometimes so significant that the malady produced was almost exclusively confined to tropical or torrid regions of the Earth' is important, but should be seen as more applicable to the period before the impact of the universalizing programmes of hospital medicine and sanitary science around the middle of the century.[25] In this context the special diseases of the tropics are best seen as analogous diseases of other special environments: jail fever, urban epidemics and hospital diseases, or those diseases linked with particular constitutional traits: race (Irish fever), gender (puerperal fever), age (childhood fevers). In other words, the discussion of 'diseases in the tropics' as well as using the universal nosologies, also remained congruent to medical geography and the diathetic notions that were still the common currency in European medicine.[26]

From Miasmas to Malaria

Any discussion of malaria in the nineteenth century has to begin with the differentiation of malaria as a generic term for miasmas and miasmatic diseases and its subsequent restriction to a specific, febrile disease. This change occurred after 1850 in the context of the general differentiation and re-designation of zymotic diseases into specific syndromes on grounds of symptomology, pathological anatomy and eventually aetiology. How quickly this occurred is a moot point for the editor of the 1883 edition of Parkes's *Manual* still used the term 'malaria' in the miasmatic sense and saw no need to alter the much-quoted phrase 'when a clime is called "unhealthy" in many cases it is simply meant that it is malarious'.[27] In Britain 'ague' still had some currency, but the preferred terms for the syndrome we can retrospectively identify as malaria were increasingly those of intermittent, remittent or paroxysmal fevers.[28] Often malaria as the exciting cause was discussed quite independently of clinical and pathological accounts of its effects in the different fevers.[29] By the early 1890s, those advancing germ explanations referred back to earlier views of malaria as having been in 'chaos'.[30] Obviously this is poor history from our perspective, though typical of the polemic that surrounded the establishment of new models of disease at this time. While there had certainly been differences of opinion about malaria in the 1860s and 1870s, these were quite typical of medicine and similar to uncertainties about many others diseases. A more insightful reading of this statement is that much of the 'chaos' had been created by the search for a germ pathology and aetiology. First, the insistence on single rather than multiple causes forced people to choose between alternatives; and, second, as such an obvious zymotic candidate as the malaria resisted easy enrolment into the canon of germ afflictions.

Before germs, remittent and intermittent fevers were either viewed as a zymotic disease produced by malarious conditions, or febrile syndromes produced by the effects of heat on the constitution – the 'chill theory'.[31] By no means were these fevers seen as a special problem of the tropics, being common in Europe and North America, especially in marshes, low-lying areas and other locations.[32] However, they were recognized as having been more prevalent in temperate regions in earlier centuries; so one implication drawn was that they had declined with the advance of civilization, or more particularly, with sanitary reform.[33] Contemporaries recognized that these fevers became both more prevalent and virulent as one moved south, though whether this was because of the greater heat or humidity, sanitary 'backwardness', or some combination of these, was the subject of debate. The important point, as evident in Hirsch's influential *Geographical and Historical Pathology*, was the continuum and the gradient of increasing incidence and intensity.[34]

Sanitarians and others supposed that a malarious poison or ferment, developing from decaying matter in the soil, was spread by evaporation after rain, or arose from soil disturbed by agricultural or urban development.[35] Such notions meant that malaria was easily assimilated to Pettenkofer's soil contamination and soil water ideas of the development of epidemic diseases.[36] Like other zymotic poisons, the malarial agent could be both a predisposing cause, weakening the system, and an exciting cause, directly precipitating disease after the poison had entered the system. In the 1850s the poisons or ferments were thought to be chemicals and lack of success in finding, let alone identifying, them was blamed on the absence of systematic chemical investigation. Some thought that the subtlety and transient quality of the principles meant their isolation would remain impossible, but few doubted their reality because of the clear and consistent effects they produced.[37] Other claims were made about the poison of malaria and these largely followed broader shifts in the explanation of zymotic diseases. Due to the association with marshes and soil conditions fungal theories had some support, especially in the United States.[38] However, Aitken noted in 1880 that no one had yet seen 'malarious spores' and his indifference to the importance of finding this 'subtle, invisible, imponderable element' is noteworthy.[39]

In the 'chill theory' the disease was defined by its symptoms – fever – not the aetiological conditions of its development. The novelty of the chill theory was the suggestion that it was not extremes of heat and humidity that were important, but the degree of variation and rates of change on the individual's physiology. As W. J. Moore confidently stated in 1881, 'experience had taught that hot days and cold nights are certain to produce fever'. Thus, Europeans either succumbed immediately or were progressively weakened before final breakdown.[40] Again, it was possible to combine the miasmatic and chill theories by supposing that internal, structural changes were first produced by an external agent, but that later attacks could 'be brought on by such causes as cold or dietetic errors'.[41] The influence of both the poison and chill theories can be seen in the three main ways of avoiding or combating the disease: 1) to find or create settlements in areas free from the poison or from extremes of temperature; 2) to take individual precautions to mitigate exposure to the same variables; and 3) to use quinine as a preventive and a cure, this acting either as an antidote to the poison or a febrifuge.[42]

In 1879 in the vogue for bacteria that followed the debates on germs from the mid-1860s and more especially Koch's work on anthrax, a disease also linked to soil contamination, Klebs and Tommasi-Crudeli claimed to have isolated the germ of malaria, a sporule-forming organism they termed *Bacillus malariae.*[43] They were authoritative figures and their account of the malarial agents was convincing. It was soon confirmed by other workers and specimens of the bacillus were shown at the Annual Meeting of the British Medical Association in 1881.[44] Italian work continued, linking bacteriological work to the clinical experience of the disease and to its epidemiology. In 1880 Laveran offered a different germ, *Oscillaria malariae,* a protozoan organism that developed in the blood of sufferers.[45] Initially this attracted far less attention, largely because Laveran was a marginal, military medical officer and was not connected to German pathology or the Pastorian network. That this germ was not a bacterium caused no immediate comment.[46] At this time, when a number of different pathogenic organisms were being identified, the limits of germs or bacteria were not considered, no possibility – animal, vegetable or mineral – had been ruled out.[47]

Smith and Sandford have discussed in detail the pathological and technical debates over the status of these two agents, and how Laveran's germ won the day.[48] However, there was also a larger cultural change as the identification of a causal agent, whatever it was, revived the flagging fortunes of the term 'malaria' and shifted the balance from a symptomatic to an aetiological definition of the disease. The response of the wider medical community to the proposed new agents was mixed. By far the largest grouping were probably unaware of any controversy; certainly few medical textbooks changed their accounts of malaria over the 1880s and if a germ was mentioned at all, it was usually tacked on to an otherwise unaltered discussion of symptomology and miasmatic conditions.[49] Laboratory findings did not have the same authority as clinical experience. Among those who were interested three different reactions can be identified. Those working in public health favoured the bacterial theory, as did the Italian school. As Tommasi-Crudeli explained to the International Medical Congress in 1884, the idea of a bacterium or 'vegetable parasite' fitted with the aetiological and epidemiological evidence that any causal organism developed in the soil and was transmitted by air or water.[50] Laveran's animal parasite impressed pathologists and laboratory workers, particularly after Richard reported in 1882 that he had found the organism in nearly 90 per cent of clinically diagnosed cases.[51] Pathologists had gained a foothold in the study of malaria when changes in the blood had been adopted in diagnosis and the presence of pigments in the spleen and liver taken as a post-mortem sign. A third group continued to doubt the existence of any germ. This consisted mainly of clinicians and public health officials in India, who were geographically and professionally remote from the new pathology, though not unaware of its claims.[52] Many felt they had already recast malaria in modern scientific and physiological terms as a paroxysmal fever, rescuing it from the vagaries of the sanitarians and miasmatists.[53]

Until the late 1880s there were no agreed criteria for establishing aetiologies. Koch's now famous postulates were slow to emerge, let alone be accepted as standards.[54] The attribution of causal relations between a specific germ and a disease syndrome usually rested on two factors: 1) the repeated presence of any organism in sufferers; and 2) the plausibility of suggested links between aetiological factors and pathological findings and the clinical experience of the disease. Demonstrating the presence of any organism was far from easy, and even when new techniques and dyes made organisms easier to see, there remained the objection that such methods created artefacts and only allowed observation of dead creatures.[55] With regard to malaria such issues concerned a relatively small group of workers in Italy and France, though their work was published in the important German journals and seems to have been read by experimental pathologists and others in Britain.[56]

In Italy, where malaria was endemic and resurgent around Rome, and where the research effort was strongest, there was an abrupt switch from the bacillus to the Laveran parasite in 1885–6.[57] The work of Richard, Golgi and Marchiafava in linking the life cycle of the protozoan to the clinical syndrome was crucial.[58] Richard showed experimentally that the protozoan was killed by quinine. He also suggested that the main pathogenic change was the alteration of red blood corpuscles by the parasites, which made them less elastic and the blood more viscous, leading to the obstruction of the circulation and, eventually, fever. The final destruction of red corpuscles could explain both the characteristic anaemia and the marked pigmentation in the spleen and liver at post-mortem. However, the work of

Marchiafava and Golgi was even more persuasive. They elaborated the life cycle of the plasmodium, linking various phases of its development to the periodicity of the fevers, and speculated further that different species of parasite might be responsible for the clinically distinct quartan and tertian forms of the disease. Pathological elaboration was a mixed blessing, as identification of the plasmodium became both more refined and more difficult. A whole series of developmental stages of the parasite were described: in 1885 some 47 forms were illustrated and by the early 1890s there were almost 200.[59] Although the organisms were difficult to handle and identify, after initiation into the methods the new observations were repeatable, which had not been the case with the bacterial claims.[60]

While enthusiastic and competent pathologists, like Welch, Councilman and Osler in the United States, were fascinated by the protozoan and were able to reproduce Italian findings, there were new obstacles to its acceptance. In the late 1880s the delineation and growing currency of Koch's postulates set more exacting standards of aetiological proof. Osler noted in 1887 that only one postulate had been met for malaria – the presence of the parasite.[61] No one had been able to meet the two other requirements: to grow the organism outside the body, and to produce malaria experimentally by the introduction into a healthy animal of isolated organisms. There were reports of the disease being produced by the inoculation of whole blood taken from sufferers, though such results lacked precision and were difficult to replicate.[62]

In Europe, the fact that the malaria pathogen was a protozoan with a complex life cycle raised no issues as to its status as a germ. Discussions of malaria were an integral part, technically and cognitively, of the development of microscopic pathology and bacteriology. Indeed, it was not uncommon to hear all the new bacterial pathogens spoken of as parasites, with the phrase 'vegetable parasites' particularly common.[63] One definition of the distinction between a zymotic and parasitic disease had been whether or not the pathogenic agent was derived from the human body.[64] Parasitic diseases were said to be due to independent animal or vegetable organisms finding a suitable place to develop on, or in, the human body, whereas zymotic diseases involved agents (chemicals, ferments) that produced some transformation of tissues, cells or molecules of the human body in their propagation. Both spontaneous generation and the theory in which the 'germs' of disease were respectively new or degraded cells (bioplasm) also assumed that disease could arise in the human body. Hence, the idea that germs were independent bacteria or other organisms, put such pathogens closer to worms and protozoa than to zymotic poisons or other matter.[65] In these terms, an important goal of the new bacteriology was to convert all zymotic diseases to parasitic, germ ones.[66]

However, in North America there was discussion of the fact that the malaria pathogen was an animal rather than a vegetable parasite, though a parasite nonetheless.[67] The solution to this problem, adopted by Osler, was to link malaria with helminth diseases, like filariasis, and with veterinary diseases where worms and flukes were more common. Some early histories of germs listed Manson's early work on filariasis, where he showed the disease to be produced by a mosquito-borne worm, as a 'germ discovery'.[68] In such contexts, protozoa were large germs and worms giant germs. It should be remembered that the meaning of bacteria, strictly rod-shaped organisms, was being extended to cover spirilla, cocci and other micro-organisms of varying shape and size, some of which might well be ultra-microscopic.

Some doctors, especially those in the tropics or with tropical experience, who had less opportunity and inclination to engage with the new pathology, were unimpressed by the germ findings about malaria.[69] For example, W. J. Moore, author of several authoritative texts on disease in India, pointed to numerous problems.[70] Malarial fevers often arose within half an hour of arrival in the tropics – could any microbe diffuse and act so rapidly? The supposed germs had not been found in the environment, so how did they spread? One opinion in India was that if malaria did exist as an entity it was water-borne, hence repeated failures to find anything in soil and water, which had yielded such a rich flora and fauna in recent cholera investigations, was damning in their eyes. In addition, the Laveran germs were never found in 100 per cent of sufferers. A study in Bombay by Vandyke Carter in 1887 found parasites in only 43 per cent of cases. Even the converts to the germ pathology reserved microscopic work for research and to confirm diagnoses made by signs and symptoms.[71] Moore also asked, what was to be made of sufferers without the germs? How could any microbe theory account for secondary attacks or breakdowns – did these remarkable organisms remain dormant and hidden for months, even years? Besides, why did one need all this talk of germs when there was a perfectly satisfactory explanation of malaria in the chill theory and the 'operation of heat on the system'. There was more at stake here than aetiology: the very nature of malaria was at issue. Moore was among those who wished to abolish the category altogether and only talk about paroxysmal, febrile diseases.[72] Appeals that all the leading pathologists in Europe and North America now accepted the *Plasmodium* cut no ice with the objectors and their long, often personal, experience of fevers.[73]

In the early 1890s discussions of malaria were typical of all diseases where a germ pathology had been shown or was suspected, except in two areas – transmission and immunity. Interest and work on the mechanisms of transmission of micro-organisms had grown, as there was a move away from 'germs-in-the-air' and 'germs everywhere' views. The preference of Pasteur, Lister and other British workers for 'free-floating' germs gave way to German ideas of fixed exchange mechanisms. Hence, the water supply, sewers, food, milk and bodily discharges all came under suspicion as conduits for germs, as did cats, dogs, birds and insects as germ carriers. The silence over the transmission of malaria covered the repeated failures to find the protozoan or its 'spores' outside the body. Thus, Davidson's review of knowledge of the disease in 1894, while fully accepting its infective and parasitic nature, could offer nothing more than a listing of factors associated with the development of the disease: soil humidity and disturbance, configuration of the country, geology, meteorology, the age, sex and profession of sufferers, and race.[74] He did not mention the speculation that insects spread the disease, either accidentally through picking up poisonous matter from the soil, or more fantastically, that blood-sucking species of insects disseminated the disease, either directly through biting or accidentally by contaminating water supplies or the soil after their death.[75] Yet, the repeated failure to demonstrate air or water conduction made mosquito transmission more plausible. A suggestive model for such a mechanism was provided by the demonstration of Theobald Smith and Kilborne of an insect vector for the protozoan causing tick-borne fever in 1893.[76] Though as late as 1896, while still favouring a role for mosquitoes, Manson was disputing the need for any elaborate process of transmission for malaria and asked 'Why should we suppose that the diffusion of the malaria germ is conducted on principles different from those regulating the diffusion of other germs'?[77]

Immunological ideas and products were of tremendous symbolic and practical importance to medicine in the 1890s.[78] The relative lack of interest in immunity to malaria, like all negatives, is difficult to explain with certainty, though a number of reasons can be suggested. First, the recurrent nature of the disease implied that the body did not, and could not, build up immunity. Second, the technical problems of working with organisms that could not be cultured meant that methods like attenuation were unavailable. Third, in the colonial context, racial immunity was assumed. Europeans seemingly had little or no immunity, while the indigenous peoples of highly malarious areas were assumed to have inherited or acquired immunity.[79] It was certainly the impression among colonial medical personnel that indigenous peoples did not suffer from malaria as much or as severely as Europeans.[80] Counter-evidence to this was cited in the medical press, but it is now clear that colonial medical practitioners had very little knowledge of the health of non-Europeans and spoke as much from ignorance as prejudice.[81] That Italian workers, dealing with malaria among their own people, did take up natural and artificial immunity, would seem to confirm the importance of the racial factor.[82]

Despite these problems, malaria was successfully enrolled as a germ disease in the 1890s, with Manson in particular promoting the position that 'Malaria is the same ... as any other germ [disease]'.[83] The growing influence in metropolitan medical circles of pathologists and the new 'bacteriologists' was a key factor in the closure upon the protozoan pathogen. The defenders of other accounts were remote geographically and marginal professionally. More and more investigators and clinicians were literally able to see the parasite as the techniques of the new pathology improved, became standardized, and were more widely diffused through medical education. Furthermore, the category of fever had less and less nosological significance and came to be regarded as a secondary effect that required to be explained in terms of an exciting pathological or physiological cause. Laboratory-generated knowledge had gained in authority due to the progressive incorporation of zymotic and other diseases to germ accounts. Few now doubted that malaria would also succumb: the only question seemed to be who, and when, would solve the outstanding questions.

What was seen to be the final piece of the puzzle, the confirmation of the insect-vector theory by Ross and Grassi in 1897, was more significant than expected. The mosquito turned out to be more than a casual or accidental carrier. Ross showed that the malaria germ went through several further developmental stages in the mosquito and was transmitted actively by inoculation both ways: from human-to-mosquito in blood, and from mosquito-to-human in the saliva of the biting insect. This made the mosquito an intermediate host as well as a vector, a role analogous to that found with entozoal diseases – e.g., snails in fluke diseases and pigs with tapeworms. The implication was that the understanding and management of this disease required zoological, even ecological, knowledge as well as medical.[84] The experience with bacteria and other germ diseases had been that what happened in the time and space between sufferers was of little moment, either because the period of time was very short, or the germ was in a dormant form. It should be remembered that part of the refutation of Pettenkofer and the latter day miasmatists had been the denial of any significant role for the environment in the development of germs. The protozoan-mosquito account now implied that the environment, albeit very differently constituted from that of the miasmatists, was all important. My suggestion is that it was only after this finding in the late 1890s that bacterial germs and protozoan and worm germs were set on different trajectories. However, these were not determined by aetiological differences on their own. They arose, too, from the way tropical medicine was institutionalized as a postgraduate specialism, and from the way malaria control policies developed.

Utilizing the New Knowledge of Malaria Transmission

The new understanding of malaria was transferred to, and gained currency in, British colonial medicine very rapidly after 1897. Its adoption was facilitated by the impetus brought to the subject by the new political interest in the health of Europeans in the tropics following the partition of Africa and the emergence of the policy of 'constructive imperialism'.[85] Those best placed to address these new concerns about the 'White Man's Grave' were metropolitan medical scientists. In Britain, the power and influence of the Indian Medical Service and its luminaries had waned, at the same time that the government and private interests behind the proposed schools of tropical medicine also ignored the expertise at the Army Medical School at Netley. In this new imperialist context, tropical diseases and malaria in particular were invested with great importance as the major impediment to the economic and political development of the tropical empire. Manson described malaria as 'by far the most important disease agency in tropical pathology' and 'the principal cause of morbidity and mortality in the tropics and sub-tropics'.[86] It was certainly the largest cause of hospitalization in India, but typhoid fever and other diseases had higher mortality rates.[87] The picture in other colonies varied, but in only a few places was malaria far and away the most serious health problem.[88] Manson's rhetoric probably had more to do with exploiting the scientific and public attention that mosquito transmission had been given, not least because it was the one germ disease where a Briton could claim a decisive discovery. The priority and significance of Ross's work was contested by Italian and French scientists, but this only served to embolden British claims.

Using the new knowledge of malarial transmission became a political goal at several levels. Practically, it suggested weak points in the cycle of transmission that could be targeted to preserve European lives. Medically, it was used to stake out new professional territory, while scientifically it engaged the Royal Society in research organization and brought the prestige of a Nobel Prize. Politically, it was used as propaganda in the promotion of a more optimistic vision of the colonial empire by Colonial Secretaries from Chamberlain onwards.

While it proved relatively easy to find the external resources to support new medical institutions, it proved more difficult to convince the medical community of the need for a new specialism and of the distinctiveness of tropical pathology.[89] In his attempts to legitimate tropical medicine as a specialism, Manson made malaria the paradigmatic 'tropical disease'. Having been an integral part of the development of germ ideas and practices for several decades, and having played a role in allowing the entry of protozoa and worms into germ discourses, malaria now became the basis for the separation of bacteria from other parasites. Manson proposed a distinction between those (parasitic/tropical) diseases that were dependent upon a geographically specific vector for their spread, with cosmopolitan (bacterial) diseases, that were spread independently of any environmental factor.[90] The idea is reasonable enough, but it does not define a special category of uniquely tropical diseases. An obvious problem was malaria where, Ross apart, all the important work had been carried out in North Africa, Italy and other locations north of the Tropic of Cancer. The *Anopheles* mosquito was also quite cosmopolitan. On the other hand, several well-known bacterial diseases, like typhoid fever, were by then more serious in the tropics than anywhere else. Manson had moved quickly from a position where all 'diseases in the tropics' would turn out to be caused by germs and for which climate was irrelevant, to one where a special group of 'tropical diseases' was caused by a unique group of pathogens and spread by intermediate host vectors, whose distribution was influenced by climate. The universality of germ theories, which had recently been so useful in attacking sanitarians and advocates of the 'chill theory', was abandoned in the rush to found the new specialism. Even if medical opposition had been stronger, there must be doubts about its ability to halt a bandwagon that enjoyed such powerful political and economic support. Moreover, in the short term Manson was vindicated as the parasite-vector model was successfully applied to redefine yellow fever, sleeping sickness and later bilharzia, and to find new diseases like Chagas' disease and the leishmaniases.[91] Institutionally, the growth of the colonial civil service and opportunities for private practice in the colonies guaranteed a steady stream of students to postgraduate courses, while imperial governments and other interests provided money for expeditions and research. In 1907, Manson reflected that 'tropical disease' was not a scientific category, but one that was 'useful and practical'.[92]

The practical context of the transfer of germ work and practices to colonial medicine from the 1890s was quite clearly to try to make the tropics healthier for the administrators, traders and experts pursuing 'constructive imperialism'. The Schools provided the theoretical knowledge and practical skills, additional to that provided in Britain and elsewhere, that a medical graduate needed to be an effective doctor in the tropics.[93] With regard to malaria, the first consequence was to reinforce quinine prophylaxis and treatment, with its action now firmly that of an 'internal disinfectant', or what Ehrlich termed a 'magic bullet'. For the other tropical diseases there was nothing similar immediately to hand, so the established advice on hygiene and constitutional management remained. Over the next decade or so, however, the treatment of tropical/parasitic diseases did see the adoption of chemotherapy (e.g., atoxyl in sleeping sickness and antimony tartrate in bilharzia) to a greater extent than with other infectious diseases, a situation which only served to reinforce a pathogen-centred construction of these diseases.[94]

The parasite-vector model was primarily interpreted as offering more to malaria prevention and control than treatment. Much of this was formalized in 'tropical hygiene', a set of practices that broke with the earlier policy of directly transferring European sanitary approaches to the overseas empire, though this is not to say that it was unaffected by trends in European public health. In the 1880s, the classical sanitarian approach of focusing on the prevention of a broad spectrum of diseases and controlling these by large-scale environmental changes (e.g., drainage, sewerage, water supplies) was both supplemented and challenged by new concerns. Preventive policies switched: 1) to targeting specific diseases; 2) to attacking such diseases in and immediately around individuals; and 3) to using disinfection to destroy pathogens directly and isolation to prevent the spread of germs from person-to-person. To a large degree this re-definition and re-direction of effort was shaped by germ theories.[95] However, other factors, like the medical takeover of public health, ideas of disease specificity, and quarantine measures to control epidemics played their part.[96]

In the late 1890s the cutting edge of public health work shifted again, from the control of disease to the promotion of health. This change was symbolized by the development of 'preventive medicine' and the provision of personal health services, like infant and maternal welfare, school medical services and wider health education, as in anti-tuberculosis campaigns. The aim now was additionally to build up the strength of people so that they could resist disease and lead healthy, productive lives, and to encourage people to feel and take responsibility for their own health.[97] This change also had diverse origins, not least in attempts by the state to promote the well-being of the mass of their population in the context of imperialism, and as a response to 'pressure from below' for reforms resulting from the extension of the franchise and the rise of socialism. The influence of germ ideas was also apparent in what one doctor called the growing evidence of 'the powers of natural resistance, or the personal factor in disease of microbic origin'.[98] The suggestion that germ pathologies helped foster a period 'when the socio-economic and political circumstances of the population had become largely irrelevant to the practice of medicine' is clearly wrong.[99] Germ theories of disease had always gone hand in hand with germ theories of health, how and why the 'soil' of some people could resist the 'seeds' of disease; a situation that had long been linked to social class, economic level and morality. If certain kinds of medical work did ignore the socio-economic position of the people, then this has to be explained, it cannot be assumed to flow directly from germ theories.

The influence of sanitarianism on colonial medical practice in the third quarter of the nineteenth century has been discussed earlier and this persisted, often in an unreformed way, well into the twentieth century and was evident in continuing advice on healthy locations. However, tropical hygiene was largely built upon variations on the policies of disinfection and isolation that had come to the fore in Europe in the 1880s. What was not immediately embraced, despite the tropical medicine being scientifically advanced and supported by reform-minded politicians, was the new preventive medicine. It could be argued that there was an inevitable time-lag between the implementation of policies in Britain and their transfer to colonial medicine, but this is unconvincing. There had been no time-lag earlier with sanitarianism, so why should there be one later when communication was more rapid and the flow of medical knowledge stronger? Besides, the notion of time-lags can be teleological, suggesting in this case that public health had to follow an inevitable path. What I want to suggest is that the form and timing of transfers involved choices. Hence, tropical hygiene selectively adopted and adapted aspects of disinfection and isolation practices and ignored other possibilities.

The main policy recommendation drawn from the parasite-vector model was to try to break the cycle of transmission by isolation practices, though not the British system of hospitals to isolate sufferers. Instead two approaches were followed: first, the isolation of healthy individuals from vectors by the use of screening and netting; and second, the isolation, or more accurately segregation, of communities and individual homes from dangerous vector-infested areas and from the indigenous population, who were now portrayed as dangerous reservoirs and carriers of disease.[100] Individual isolation was relatively cheap and eminently suitable for Europeans and wealthy indigenes, while medically endorsed segregation legitimated and reinforced other prejudices. Disinfection policies concentrated on attacking both the *Plasmodium* and *Anopheles.* Koch recommended attacking the protozoan with quinine, administered to sufferers identified in mass blood screenings, while British doctors put greater stress on the control of mosquitoes, which seemed more obvious and tangible targets.[101] Ross touted the complete extirpation of the mosquito, while Manson concentrated on breaking contact between mosquitoes and humans.[102] This vector-focused approach was developed for other diseases, e.g., yellow fever and sleeping sickness, and had a very visible public relations success in Gorgas's work during the construction of the Panama Canal.[103] However, such relatively simple solutions were soon found wanting and by the 1910s a much more complex, if not perplexing, understanding of the disease, mosquito ecology and control possibilities had built up.[104]

However, important features of the 'isolation/disinfection' strategy became entrenched, with a number of intended and unintended consequences. First, it established the idea of seeing tropical regions in terms of the threat posed by a single disease and targeting one disease at a time for control.[105] Second, the focus on the parasite, vector and transmission, at the expense of immunity, educational programmes and self-help, defined malaria as a zoological and ecological problem rather than a medical one. Third, relatedly, the 'vertical' approaches that became so characteristic of malaria control meant that little investment was made in 'horizontal' health protection and promotion agencies. Fourth, tropical medicine was maintained in a relatively marginal position in world medicine, with strong links to biology and ecology, and that its differences with 'temperate' theory and practice, rather than its similarities, were emphasized. It was not, therefore, that the socio-economic conditions were ignored, rather that there was a deliberate choice to reject such determinants of health and to regard the indigenous peoples of tropical countries as passive victims rather than as actors who could play a part in health programmes. John Farley recently put the same point in a different way, when he termed the twentieth-century medical effort for the Third World as 'imperial tropical medicine'. This was in terms of the 'definition' and 'imposition' of policies by colonial and post-colonial agencies, and the consequent 'non-involvement' of the indigenous population.[106]

Conclusion

While I would not want to place too much emphasis on words, it does seem to me that the shift in terminology from 'disease in the tropics' to 'tropical diseases' was significant.[107] The former signalled that the understanding and management of diseases in the tropics was contiguous with that of other diseases, and that medical practitioners saw any differences between diseases as of degree rather than kind. Thus, during the search for the germs of 'diseases in the tropics' from the 1870s, it was fully expected that the specific agents causing tropical fevers would turn out to be just like those being found to cause fevers in Europe. Indeed, the capture of malaria, the greatest of all sanitarian evils, by the germists was one of their greatest triumphs. So it was only from the late 1890s that significant attempts were made to shift malaria into distinct discourses devoted to a new class of parasitic, tropical diseases. These were based on a purportedly unique association between tropical diseases, animal parasites and vector transmission of disease – the essence of what we now know as Mansonian tropical medicine. Thus, the transformation of malaria into a tropical disease was not simply a consequence of the decline in its incidence in Britain and Europe, but due to the re-designation of a disease that had been central to zymotic and germ discourses from the 1840s to the 1890s. Crucially, the new tropical medicine gained both a separate social base and credibility from the seeming success of the control practices of tropical hygiene. However, the emergence of this notion of 'tropical diseases', and of its characteristic 'vertical' disease control programmes, cannot be the attributed to the germ theory of disease *per se.* There were many ideas and actions that were and could have been derived from germ work and from the parasite-vector model. It has been argued here that the particular, and perhaps peculiar, meanings and implications of germ ideas, first adopted by Manson and then institutionalized in tropical medicine, were shaped by the micro- and macro-politics of British colonial imperialism and its medical politics.

Notes

1. H. H. Scott, *A History of Tropical Medicine* (London: Edward Arnold, 1939); W. D. Foster, *A History of Parasitology* (London: E. and S. Livingstone, 1970); and P. C. C. Garnham, *Progress in Parasitology* (London: Athlone Press, 1970).
2. M. Worboys, 'The emergence of tropical medicine', in G. Lemaine *et al* (eds), *Perspectives on the Emergence of New Scientific Disciplines* (Paris: Mouton, 1976), 75–89; M. Worboys, 'The emergence and early development of parasitology', in K. S. Warren and J. Z. Bowers, (eds), *Parasitology: A Global Perspective* (New York: Springer Verlag, 1983), 1–18; M. Lyons, *The Colonial Disease: A Social History of Sleeping Sickness in Northern Zaire, 1900–1940* (Cambridge: Cambridge University Press, 1991), 64–75; J. Farley, *Bilharzia: A History of Imperial Tropical Medicine* (Cambridge: Cambridge University Press, 1991), 13–30.
3. There is no recent monograph on the history of the germ theory of disease that reflects recent historical approaches and concerns. However, a number of studies suggest that the extant, often heroic, histories are inadequate. See: C. J. Lawrence and R. Dixey, 'Lister and the germ theories of disease', in C. J. Lawrence (ed.), *Medical Theory, Surgical Practice* (London: Routledge, 1992); M. Warner, 'Hunting the yellow fever germ: The principle and practice of aetiological proof in late nineteenth century America', *Bulletin of the History of Medicine,* 59 (1985), 361–82; C. Hamlin, *The Science of Impurity,* (Bristol: Adam Hilger 1990).
4. P. Manson, *Tropical Diseases: A Manual of the Diseases of Warm Climates* (London: Cassell & Co., 1898), xii; P. Manson, 'The necessity of special training in tropical medicine', *Journal of Tropical Medicine,* 2 (1897), 1–4.
5. K. S. Warren and E. F. Pursell (eds), *The Current Status of Parasitology* (New York: Josiah Macy Fdn, 1981), 1–20.
6. J. Farley, 'Parasites and the germ theory of disease' in C. E. Rosenberg and J. Golden (eds), *Framing Disease* (New Brunswick: Rutgers University Press, 1992), 45. Although Farley talks of 'parasites' and 'bacteria' never having been really discussed together, the last section of the chapter is nonetheless entitled 'The Parting of the Ways'.
7. B. Latour, *The Pasteurization of France* (Cambridge, Mass.: Harvard University Press, 1988).
8. O. Temkin, *The Double Face of Janus* (Baltimore: Johns Hopkins University Press, 1985), 436.
9. M. Worboys, 'The sanatorium treatment of consumption in Britain, 1890–1910', in J. V. Pickstone (ed.), *Medical Innovation in Historical Perspective* (London: Macmillan, 1992), 47–71.
10. Singer and Underwood observed in 1962 that, 'Tropical diseases ... form a group, not from their nature but in their mode of protection'.

C. Singer and E. A. Underwood, *A Short History of Medicine* (Oxford: Clarendon Press, 1962), 453.

11. J. Johnson, *The Influence of Tropical Climates, More Especially the Climate of India, on European Constitutions* (London: Stockdale, 1815); J. R. Martin, *The Influence of Tropical Climates on European Constitutions* (London: J. Churchill 1856): *idem, The Influence of Tropical Climates in Producing the Acute Endemic Diseases of Europeans* (London: J. Churchill, 1861, 2nd edn); J. A. Horton, *Diseases of Tropical Climates and their Treatment* (London: 1874).
12. L. G. Wilson, 'Fevers and science in early nineteenth century medicine', *Journal of the History of Medicine,* 33 (1978), 386–407.
13. W. J. Moore, *Health in the Tropics; or the sanitary art as applied to Europeans in India* (London: J. & A. Churchill, 1862). Moore had been one of Chadwick's correspondents in 1844, reporting on Nottingham for the sanitary inquiry into the condition of large towns in 1846.
14. D. N. Livingstone, 'Human acclimatization: Perspectives on a contested field of inquiry in science, medicine and geography', *History of Science,* 25 (1987), 359–94; M. Harrison, '"The tender frame of man": Medical men and the acclimatisation question, 1760–1840', paper given to the conference of *Disease and Society in the Developing World: Exploring New Perspectives,* 24–6 September, 1992, College of Physicians of Philadelphia.
15. P. D. Curtin, *Death by Migration: Europe's Encounter with the Tropical World in the Nineteenth Century* (Cambridge: Cambridge University Press, 1989), 1–39.
16. J. V. Pickstone, 'Dearth, dirt and fever epidemics: Rewriting the history of British "public health", 1750–1850', in P. Slack and T. Ranger (eds), *Epidemics and Ideas,* (Oxford: Oxford University Press, 142.
17. D. Arnold, 'Cholera and colonialism in British India', *Past and Present,* 113 (1986), 118–51.
18. Royal Commission on the Sanitary State of the Army in India, 1863, Parliamentary Papers, 1863 [3184], xix, 1.
19. D. Arnold, 'Medical priorities and practice in nineteenth century British India', *South Asia Research,* 5 (1985), 167–83.
20. M. Harrison, 'Tropical medicine in nineteenth century India', *British Journal for the History of Science,* 25 (1992), 312.
21. E. Parkes, *Manual of Practical Hygiene* (London: J. & A. Churchill, 1864), 548, 551 and 559.
22. *Ibid.,* 521. In this context Parkes was talking of malaria in the sense of poisonous air, not the specific disease. The problem was that 'air' was the most difficult medium to alter or control by sanitary measures.
23. J. Notter (ed.), *Parkes' Manual of Practical Hygiene* (London: J. & A. Churchill 1891), 643.
24. Curtin, *op. cit.* (note 15), 104–58.
25. Harrison, *op. cit.* (note 20), 305.

26. E. Ackerknecht, *History and Geography of the Most Important Diseases* (New York: 1965); C. E. Rosenberg, *Explaining Epidemics and other Studies in the History of Medicine* (Cambridge: Cambridge University Press, 1992), 9–32.
27. F. S. B. de Chaumont (ed.), *Parkes' Manual of Practical Hygiene* (London: J. & A. Churchill, 1883), 339.
28. J. Bristowe, *A Treatise on the Theory and Practice of Medicine* (London: Smith Elder, 1876 1st edn), 276–87.
29. W. Aitken, *The Science and Practice of Medicine* (London: Chas. Griffin & Co. 1880, 7th edn), Vol. I. The nature of malaria and of the malarious fevers (419–42) was discussed quite separately from ague and remittent fevers (665–78).
30. British Medical Journal (hereafter *BMJ*), ii (1894), 811.
31. C. F. Oldham, *What is Malaria? and Why is it most intense in Hot Climates?* (London: H.K. Lewis, 1871).
32. Aitken, *op. cit.* (note 29), (1880), Vol. II, 1105 *et seq.*
33. On the history of malaria in Europe see: L. J. Bruce Chwatt and J. de Zulueta, *The Rise and Fall of Malaria in Europe* (Oxford: Oxford University Press, 1980).
34. A. Hirsch, (trans. C. Creighton), *Handbook of Geography and Historical Pathology* (London: New Sydenham Society 1883), 197.
35. W. Aitken, *A Handbook of the Science and Practice of Medicine* (London: R. Griffin, 1858), 24–40.
36. C- E. A. Winslow, *The Conquest of Epidemic Disease: A Chapter in the History of Ideas* (Madison, Wisc.: University of Wisconsin Press, 1943), 311–36. Later there was support for what was termed the water conduction theory of transmission, where drinking water rather than the air was implicated.
37. Parkes, *op. cit.* (note 21), 254.
38. Among the most cited were: J. K. Mitchell, *Cryptogamous Origin of Malarious and Epidemic Fevers* (Philadelphia: Lea & Blanchard, 1849); J. H. Salisbury, 'On the causes of intermittent and remittent fever', *American Journal of Medical Science,* 51 (1866) 51–75. Such claims were reviewed in J. Fayrer, *On the Climate and Fevers of India* (London: J. & A. Churchill, 1882), 26–9. On malaria in North America, see: E. Ackerknecht, 'Malaria in the Upper Mississippi Valley, 1760–1900', *Bulletin of the History of Medicine,* 4 (1945), Supplement No. 1.
39. W. Aitken, *op. cit.* (note 29), (1880), Vol. II, 424.
40. W. J. Moore, 'Malaria vs. recognizable climatic influences', *Indian Medical Gazette,* 16 (1881), 293–306; W. J. Moore, 'The constitutional requirements for tropical climates', *Transactions of the Epidemiological Society of London,* 4 (1884–5), 32–51; C. F. Oldham, 'The nature and origin of climatic fevers in India [malarial]', *Transactions of the Epidemiological Society of London,* 2 (1882–3), 564–79.

41. Notter, *op. cit.* (note 23), 462.
42. On the use of quinine see: Curtin, *op. cit.* (note 15), 132–7; Cf. W. Cohen, 'Malaria and French imperialism', *Journal of African History,* 24 (1983) 23–36.
43. E. Klebs and C. Tommasi-Crudeli, *Archiv fur Experimental Pathologie,* 11 (1879), 311–98.
44. E. Marchiafava and G. Cuboni, *Archiv fur Experimental Pathologie,* 13 (1881), 31–43. *BMJ,* ii (1881) In the 1870s and early 1880s the term bacteria had yet to take on its generic meaning and only referred to rod-shaped organisms. The origin of the word was in the Greek word for a 'stick', hence in most classifications micrococci were different organisms.
45. C. L. A. Laveran, *Bulletin of the Academy of Medicine,* 9 (1880), 9: 1235; *Lancet,* ii (1881) 840–1.
46. J. Fayrer, 'Malaria', *Transactions of the Epidemiological Society of London,* 1 (1881–2), 15–25, noted in passing that Laveran's germ was 'a ciliated corpuscle'.
47. C. Flügge, (trans. W. Watson Cheyne), *Micro-organisms, with Special Reference to the Etiology of Infectious Diseases* (London: New Sydenham Society, 1880); E. M. Crookshank, *An Introduction to Practical Bacteriology,* (London: H. K. Lewis, 1886).
48. D. C. Smith and L. B. Sandford, 'Laveran's germ: The reception and use of a medical discovery', *American Journal of Tropical Medicine and Hygiene,* 34 (1985), 2–20. Also see the encyclopaedic L. J. Bruce Chwatt, 'The history of malaria from prehistory to eradication', in W. H. Wernersdorfer and I. MacGregor, *Malaria: Principles and Practice of Malariology* (London: Churchill Livingstone, 1988), 1–59.
49. Bristowe's textbook of medicine hardly altered its account of malaria between the first edition in 1876 and the seventh in 1890. J. Bristowe, *A Treatise on the Theory and Practice of Medicine,* (London: Smith Elder, 1876 1st edn; 1890 7th edn). However, Fagge's textbook of medicine mentioned the Malaria bacillus in its first edition in 1886, and from 1888 switched to what was called the *'contagium vivum'* of Laveran and Richard. C. H. Fagge (subsequent edns. with P. H. Pye Smith), A Textbook of Medicine (London: J. & A. Churchill, 1886 1st edn; 1888 2nd edn; 1891 3rd edn; 1901 4th edn).
50. C. Tommasi-Crudeli, 'La production naturelle de la malaria', *Proceedings of the International Medical Congress, Copenhagen,* 1884; *BMJ,* ii (1884), 408.
51. E. Richard, 'Sur la parasite de la malaria', *Gazette Medicale de Paris,* 4 (1882), 252; *Lancet,* i (1882), 993.
52. C. F. Oldham, 'The bacillus malariae', *Indian Medical Gazette,* 17 (1882), 63–5.
53. W. J. Moore, *BMJ,* i (1887), 986.
54. T. D. Brock, *Robert Koch: A Life in Medicine and Bacteriology* (New York: Science Tech, 1988), 179–82; Cf. W. Coleman, 'Koch's comma

bacillus: The first year', *Bulletin of the History of Medicine,* 46 (1985), 315–42.

55. Smith & Sandford, *op. cit.* (note 48), (1985), notes in one case that reported cocci might have been 'stained plasmodia, crystals of excess stain, or contaminants'.
56. See the bibliography in Crookshank, *op. cit.* (note 47), (1885), 406–7.
57. J. Mannaberg, *The Malarial Parasites* (London: New Sydenham Society, 1894), 'Historical Introduction'.
58. Smith & Sandford, *op. cit.* (note 48), 12–14.
59. P. Manson, *BMJ,* ii (1894), 1306.
60. G. M. Sternberg, *Special Report: Experimental Investigations Relating to the Etiology of Malarial Fevers* (Washington: National Board of Health, 1882), iii, 65–82. On the wider American reaction see: C. P. Russell, *Medical Record,* 24 (1883), 177–9 and 303.
61. W. Osler, *BMJ,* i (1887), 556–61.
62. *Lancet,* i (1882) 1004; also Smith & Sandford, *op. cit.* (note 48) 11.
63. For example, Aitken's 'Science and Practice of Medicine' (1880), (note 29), spoke directly of 'the bacteria group of parasites', 144–5 and discussed them in its section on 'Human Parasites' after Entozoa, Endozoa, Entophyta and Epiphyta. Also, Koch tubercle bacillus was often referred to as a 'vegetable parasite' and that he was claiming that tuberculosis was a parasitic disease. See: *BMJ,* i (1880), 23; ii (1881), 187; *Lancet,* i (1882), 694.
64. J. Simon, *Fifth Annual Report on the State of Public Health in 1863,* Parliamentary Papers, 1864 [3416] xxvii, 1. Also see Simon's contribution on 'Contagion' in Quain's *Dictionary of Medicine,* (London: 1878), where he again includes discussion of 'parasites' such as scabies, trichiniasis and other worm infections.
65. L. S. Beale, *Disease Germs: Their Nature and Origin* (London: J. & A. Churchill: 1872).
66. G. C. Henderson, 'The progress of zymotic micro-pathology', *Transactions of the Epidemiological Society of London,* 1, 1881–2, 156–74; cf. C. Creighton, *The Unconscious Memory of Disease* (London: 1884).
67. This perhaps reflected the greater strength of veterinary medicine in the United States (e.g. Osler's work on comparative pathology) and it may be that John Farley's notion of a clear distinction between parasites and germs is specific to the United States. See: V. Harden, 'Rocky Mountain spotted fever research and the development of the insect vector theory, 1900–1930', *Bulletin of the History of Medicine,* 59 (1985), 449–66.
68. A. Smart, 'A chronology of disease-germs', *BMJ,* ii (1884). The list, with dates that modern historians would question, included: Obermeier – relapsing fever (1868); Koch – anthrax (1874); Sanderson and Chauveau – vaccine germs (1869); Manson – Filaria

(1881); Eberth – typhoid fever (1881); Koch – tuberculosis (1882) and cholera (1883).

69. Fayrer, *op. cit.* (note 46), 24, noted 'The great tendency now-a-days is to trace all disease to a specific cause, but we must not lose sight of the possibility of causes developed in the body, and altered conditions of the nerve-centres and vaso-motor action, and so on, by forces influencing from without.'
70. W. J. Moore, *BMJ*, i (1887) 865.
71. H. V. Carter, *Scientific Memoirs of the Medical Officers of India*, 3 (1888), 139–67.
72. *BMJ*, ii (1895), 394, 503, 560; i (1896) 487, 696, 1135, 1217.
73. The persistence and influence of the Indian perspective was evident in 1897 with the publication of Allbutt's *System of Medicine* (London: Macmillan, 1897) Vol. II, of a chapter by Sir John Fayrer 'On the climate and some of the fevers of India', 295–352. Fayrer claimed (309f.) that the predisposing influence of climate was far more important than the new, microbial exciting causes being identified.
74. A. Davidson, *Hygiene and Disease of Warm Climates*, (Edinburgh: Young J. Pentland, 1893), 144.
75. Those who had suggested that mosquitoes had some role in the spread of the disease include: A. F. A. King, *Popular Science Monthly*, 23 (1883), 644–58; J. Nott, *New Orleans Medical and Surgical Journal*, 4 (1888), 563–901; A. Laveran, *Paludism*, ((London: New Sydenham Society, 1893). Also see the discussion in *BMJ*, i (1896) 401, 641.
76. T. Smith and F. L. Kilborne, *Investigations into the Nature, Causation, and Prevention of Southern Cattle Fever*, (Washington, D.C.: Government Printing Office, 1893). This was cited as a precedent by Bignami, *BMJ*, ii (1896), 143.
77. *Lancet*, ii (1896), 1716. Manson was opposing Bignami's idea of inoculation by mosquitoes, against his belief that the germs were spread when mosquitoes died and decomposed in soil or water. *BMJ*, i (1896), 401, 530, 641, 712, 774.
78. P. Weindling, 'From medical research to clinical practice: Serum therapy for diphtheria in the 1890s', in Pickstone, *op. cit.* (note 9), 72–83.
79. Davidson, *op. cit.* (note 74), 143
80. Manson, *op. cit.* (note 4), 103.
81. *BMJ*, i (1890); i (1892) 445, 535.
82. A. Celli, *Malaria: According to New Researches* (London: Longman Green, 1900), 103–17.
83. Manson, *Lancet*, ii (1896), 1716.
84. The second edition of Allbutt's *System of Medicine* (London: Macmillan, 1907) Vol. II, discussed malaria in a new section on tropical diseases and carried a long zoological introduction on the parasite and vector species.

85. R. V. Kubicek, *The Administration of Imperialism* (Durham, NC: Duke University Press, 1972), Ch. 6.
86. Manson, *op. cit.* (note 4), 1.
87. Parkes, *op. cit.* (note 21), (1891), 645–7.
88. Curtin, *op. cit.* (note 15), 80–103.
89. In Britain the two schools of tropical medicine opened in 1898 as independent institutions with no formal affiliation to any medical school or university. Also see: Worboys, 'Emergence of tropical medicine' (note 2), 88–9.
90. P. Manson, 'On the necessity of special education in tropical diseases', *Journal of Tropical Medicine,* 2 (1897); Farley, *op. cit.* (note 6), 42–44.
91. Worboys, 'Tropical diseases' in W. F. Bynum and R. Porter (eds), *Companion Encyclopaedia of the History of Medicine* (London: Routledge 1993), 512–36.
92. Manson, 'Introduction', Allbutt's *System,* (1907), Vol. II (ii), 1–2.
93. P. H. Manson-Bahr, *The History of the School of Hygiene and Tropical Medicine, Memoir* No. 11, (London: London School of Hygiene and Tropical Medicine, 1956).
94. M. Weatherall, *In Search of a Cure* (Oxford: Oxford University Press, 1990), 59.
95. G. Rosen, *A History of Public Health* (Baltimore: Johns Hopkins University Press, 1958; new edn 1993), 270–319.
96. E. Fee and D. Porter, 'Public health, preventive medicine, and professionalization: Britain and the United States in the nineteenth century', in A. Wear (ed.), *Medicine in Society* (Cambridge: Cambridge University Press, 1992), 249–76.
97. C. Lawrence, 'Laboratory politics', *Medical History, (*1993), 449–52; D. Porter, '"Enemies of the Race": Biology, environmentalism and public health in Edwardian Britain', *Victorian Studies,* 39 (1991), 159–78.
98. S. MacKenzie, *Transactions of the Medical Society of London,* 25, 1902 302–18.
99. Farley, *op. cit.* (note 2), 292.
100. P. Manson, Colonial Office Papers, CO 885/7, No. 129, 24 September, 1900, 43. Also see: L. Spitzer, 'The mosquito and segregation in Sierra Leone', *Canadian Journal of African Studies,* 2 (1968) 49–61; P. D. Curtin, 'Medical knowledge and urban planning in tropical Africa', *American Historical Review,* 90 (1985), 594–613; J. W. Cell, 'Anglo-Indian medical theory and the origins of segregation in West Africa', *American Historical Review,* 91 (1986) 307–35.
101. R. Koch, 'Address on Malaria', *Journal of State Medicine,* 10 (1901).
102. R. Ross, *Mosquito Brigades and How to Organise Them* (London: George Philip &Son, 1902); R. Ross, *Instructions for the Prevention of Malaria Fever for the Use of Residents in Malarious Places* (Liverpool: Liverpool School of Tropical Medicine, 1900) Memoir No. 1);

Manson, CO 885/7, No. 129, 39–40. Laveran offered similar recommendations to the French government.

103. L. Bruce Chwatt, 'Ronald Ross, William Gorgas and malaria eradication', *American Journal of Tropical Medicine and Hygiene,* 26 (1977), 1071–9.

104. J. W. W. Stephens and S. R. Christophers, *The Practical Study of Malaria and Other Blood Parasites* (London: 1903); C. W. Daniels, *Tropical Medicine and Hygiene* (London: 1913); G. Harrison, *Mosquitoes, Malaria and Man: A History of Hostilities since 1880* (London: John Murray, 1978).

105. G. Prins, 'But what was the disease? The present state of health and healing in African studies', *Past and Present* 124 (1989) 159–79.

106. Farley, *op. cit.* (note 2), 293.

107. The term 'tropical disease' was used before the late 1890s, though much less often than 'diseases of warm climates' or 'diseases in the tropics'.

10

Social Status and Imperial Service: Tropical Medicine and the British Medical Profession in the Nineteenth Century

Douglas Melvin Haynes

Historians have long explained the history of tropical medicine in terms of British overseas expansion. Since the seventeenth century, contact with the tropical world exposed Europeans to a seemingly alien disease environment. More than any single factor, the death and sickness among Europeans generated the image of the tropics as the 'White Man's Grave' and spurred investigation into the cause, prevention, and treatment of tropical disease.[1] The growth in the volume of the literature and variety of tropical diseases paralleled the growth of the tropical empire in the eighteenth and nineteenth centuries.[2] Perhaps the most explicit link between overseas expansion and tropical medicine was the decision of the British imperial state in the late nineteenth century to support and encourage schools of tropical medicine in London and Liverpool. These schools trained imperial doctors in the latest specialist knowledge and investigated endemic and epidemic diseases that threatened the political and economic health of the empire.[3]

The emphasis on overseas expansion is well-deserved. Too often, however, the stress on expansion has tended to reduce the history of tropical medicine to the mere epi-phenomenon of imperialism/ colonialism or to the inspired genius of great men, or both.[4] By overlooking other related social processes, this functional explanation has unduly reinforced the supposed distinction between the history of Britain and the history of empire. This was hardly the case. Several case studies on tropical disease have shown how the interaction between the social practice of medical-scientific investigation in the periphery and the centre – as much as the exigencies of empire – combined to shape and validate tropical disease knowledge.[5]

In this essay I want to discuss how the social position of the medical professional in general, and in the imperial services in particular, shaped the discourse about tropical medicine in the nineteenth century. For most of the century, the metropolitan profession ignored the problem of tropical disease – in large part because it was associated with low-status careers in the imperial services. After the mid-1880s, this perception changed. Overcrowding in the profession transformed tropical disease from a problem on the margins of the profession to the centre. In spite of the reputation of the services for denying medical professionals the social position thought commensurate with their education and training, career uncertainty made imperial appointments attractive as occupational safe-havens.

Overcrowding, together with imperial activity in the tropics, also sustained the first metropolitan discourse about tropical medicine. After years of indifference, the metropolitan profession 'discovered' and appropriated the problem of tropical disease. It actively promoted the need for greater official attention and resources for tropical medicine in the interest of empire. At the heart of this discourse was the social status of medical professionals in the services. If overcrowding did anything, it magnified the uneven power relationship between the services and medical professionals which underscored their historically subordinate status. Proponents of tropical medicine sought to enhance the social position of imperial doctors by tying the conquest of tropical disease to the creation of distinctive career opportunities and greater authority for medical professionals in the services.

Status anxiety dogged the medical profession. Although the profession, which included physicians, surgeons and apothecaries, rarely recruited from the higher social classes, it sought the social position and recognition of genteel society. Central to the collective social identity of practitioners was independence.[6] Whether in the eighteenth or nineteenth century, independence defined the gentleman.[7] An independent income liberated an individual from the dictates of an employer, furnished time to pursue self-directed interests, and permitted the unmediated expression of opinion. In short, an income provided autonomy.

Yet, no matter how often members of the medical profession insisted on their right to be treated as belonging to the genteel social orders, their calling placed them in a web of dependent relationships. The success of a private practice depended to a great extent on the personal confidence of patients and their willingness to pay for services rendered. It could be argued that public positions in voluntary hospitals, the various state services, such as the Poor Law and Prison Medical Services, or contracted services with friendly societies, diminished the dependence of doctors on paying patients. Admittedly, these positions did provide a steady income, a degree of visibility, and potentially useful social networks for doctors hoping to launch their careers in private practice. But, dependence on a salary or contract fees simply illustrated the humble social origins of medical professionals. Moreover, the power of lay supervisors of public institutions to control salary and fees, particularly during periods of overcrowding, vitiated the voice of medical men in shaping their official duties and responsibilities.[8]

The sense of dependence and powerlessness was regarded as being far worse in the services. Over the course of the century, the imperial service attracted many doctors, especially those born either in Scotland or Ireland, who lacked the necessary economic and social resources to establish a practice in London – the centre of the profession – much less in their native lands. In fact, Irish and Scottish doctors were represented far out of proportion to their share of the population of the United Kingdom.[9] In the Army Medical Department, they accounted for nearly three-quarters of all medical officers, and 60 per cent of medical officers in the three services (that is Bengal, Bombay and Madras), that made up the Indian Medical Service between 1860 and 1895. Of the 482 surgeons joining the Royal Navy between 1870 and 1880, 52 per cent were born in Ireland, 26 per cent in Scotland and 21 per cent in England.[10]

Besides restricted occupational opportunities, other factors undermined the social position of medical professionals in the imperial services. Multi-year pledges of service and the prohibition against public criticism by service personnel effectively gagged imperial doctors. As a social organization, the officer corps of the British Army and the Royal Navy was anything but egalitarian. Service culture and regulations buttressed the social status of officers who were typically the younger sons of the landed classes and members of the prosperous middle classes.[11] *Punch,* the satirical periodical, mordantly described the qualifications of prospective army surgeons in the House Guards in a mock advertisement:

> In addition to their professional qualifications, they must possess a capacity of being continually and contentedly Snubbed, and patiently submitting to any amount of Insult. They will be required at the mess table to occupy a position subordinate to that of every combatant officer, even the youngest Ensign, whose permission it will be

> necessary for them to ask for the purpose of giving the band or the attendants any kind of order... No Thin-Skinned Persons, endowed with any Self-Respect whatever, or animated in the least degree by Feelings of a Gentleman, need apply.[12]

In a similar vein, the author of a report on the high rate of turnover in the Colonial Medical Service of the British West Indies deplored the 'harsh and unworthy conduct of superior officials'. Colonial authorities were warned that 'Honourable and educated gentlemen may be willing to risk their life at the call of duty, but they will never submit to be bullied or cajoled'.[13]

As many imperial doctors were wont to complain, the services were the last place to be treated like a 'gentleman'.[14] In pamphlets, letters to the medical press, and guides, they condemned a system that ignored their training, compelled them to languish as junior officers indefinitely, and reduced them to clients when seeking promotion. Menial tasks, such as branding and the obligation to monitor corporal punishment, were found distasteful. The blatant preference given to officers in the distribution of sick-leave, cabin quarters, and order of precedence on public occasions were bitter reminders of their subordinate status.[15]

Neither royal warrants under the hand of the Secretary of State for War nor orders-in-council promulgated by the Lords of the Admiralty furnished relief. To be fair, administrative action throughout the period led to improved pay and liberalized pension rules.[16] Nevertheless, these reforms rarely redressed the status grievances of imperial doctors. The medical press excoriated the Government of India, the House Guards, and the Lords of the Admiralty for either wilfully ignoring or withholding the assimilation of relative rank, that is equivalent rank for equal time served, and other signs of official recognition.[17]

Nor did the metropolitan campaign to improve the social position of doctors in the services necessarily elevate the esteem of public service. Proponents of service reform sought to browbeat the services into improving conditions by pointing to the excess of vacancies over candidates.[18] They, too, adopted a rhetoric of reform that played up national and class stereotypes. A career decision, rather than referring to the importance of social and economic resources in occupational success in the British medical profession, jeopardized one's social credibility as a medical officer. Medical students were discouraged from accepting a stipend from the Lords of the Admiralty as an incentive to serve in the Royal Navy:

> Men who could accept such humiliating terms could not expect to be received on terms of equality by officers who value themselves for their independence, their professional honour, and their attainments. The seamen themselves are not without discernment; and such a class of officers of bond, if imported into the service, could never either command confidence or respect.[19]

Still worse, the relative absence of middle-class English medical graduates compromised the professional integrity of the services. A note on the list of candidates who passed the examination into the Army Medical Department in 1864 denounced the Director-General of the Department:

> The small number of candidates for the appointments, the enormous prevalence of the Hiberian element, and the almost total absence of English students, are as remarkable on this occasion as on former occasions. This is a list which the Director-General must feel shame in presenting to the English profession: it shows emphatically the profound unpopularity of the Department over which he presides. [20]

The effect of self-respecting English medical graduates preferring civilian careers was compared to Gresham's Law, and led to low-class and unaccomplished Scottish and Irish surgeons 'swamping' the ranks of the services.[21]

Imperial doctors, owing to their tour of duty in the tropics and their charge to look after the health of service personnel, made the problem of tropical disease their own special concern. It was, however, this very connection between low-status imperial service careers and tropical medicine that consigned the problem of tropical disease to the margins of interest of the metropolitan profession for several decades. Of course, the geographical distance between the so-called temperate and tropical worlds minimized the immediate relevance of tropical medicine. Nonetheless, then as today, the prestige which invests problem areas in medicine is shaped as much by the social meaning of illness as by the social position of practitioners within the profession and society at large.[22]

Hence, the difficulty Joseph Fayrer, a graduate of Edinburgh University and medical officer in the Bengal Medical Service, had in trying to fathom why there was so little interest in tropical surgery in the West appears slightly disingenuous.[23] The same can be said of William Campbell MacLean who justified the need for his lectures on tropical diseases at the Army Medical School by pointing to the lack of time and clinical resources of the metropolitan medical schools.[24] Metropolitan indifference to tropical medicine was not symptomatic of the over-taxed time commitments of the profession in general nor the limited resources of medical schools in particular, but, rather, was due to status priorities. Indifference simply reflected the fact that imperial service was not a preferred career.

Imperial doctors did not simply accept their occupational marginality within the profession and in the services. Many attempted to enhance their occupational position by privileging their specialist understanding of tropical disease and health. It is important to note that the growing volume of tropical medicine publications in the nineteenth century was not necessarily intended to redefine medicine *per se.* In fact, metropolitan theory and practice also related disease in the temperate world to the operation of the environment as distinct from a specific pathogen.[25] Rather, imperial doctors sought to situate the authority of tropical medicine in themselves by distinguishing their occupational experience in the periphery from the centre.

Stewart Henderson, an army surgeon who received his medical degree from King's College in Aberdeen, criticized the Army Board's decision to appoint only doctors with a diploma from the exclusive College of Physicians to such lucrative and prestigious posts as army hospital physician and physician to regimental forces. Henderson complained that this preference deprived soldiers of the skill and knowledge of surgeons who were familiar with diseases of the hot climates.[26] In a letter to the Secretary of State for War, Andrew Halliday, the Edinburgh-trained Deputy Inspector-General for Hospitals in the British West Indies, emphasized that no matter how well educated young recruits might be or 'deep read in the theory of physic, they can have but little practical experience in the treatment of any class of diseases even in Europe, and certainly none of those that are common within the tropics'.[27] W. J. Moore, Honorary Surgeon to the Viceroy of India, objected to the 'absurdity and fallacy of the supposition that the practitioners of one clime can safely prescribe for the diseases of another'.[28]

Norman Chevers, a graduate of Glasgow University, cautioned newly arrived doctors in India to divest

> the mind of a host of strong opinions – such as that the medical man should never leave his house without his case of bleeding lancets, that colchicams is 'good' for rheumatism, that mercury is supreme in hepatic diseases, and that cathartics are therapeutic agents of almost Morisonian universality.[29]

Patrick Manson, a graduate of the University of Aberdeen and medical officer in the Imperial Chinese Customs Service, in his 1884 presidential address to the Hong Kong Medical Society remarked:

> The lay mind abandoned the 'Jos Sedley' and 'Naboob' type; but, alas, the profession is for once behind the age – it sticks to its traditions. Anyone who has been through the Suez Canal is assumed in London consulting rooms to have an enlarged or otherwise diseased liver; that he eats and drinks too much; and that he stands in need of blue pills, nitro-nuriatic acid and quinine.[30]

A standard refrain in tropical medical texts was the need for lay and military officials to submit to the expertise of doctors. Of the dire consequences of ignoring medical expertise, Robert Jackson, an army surgeon who, against regulation, was appointed to head a hospital in the British West Indies, wrote that 'the ravage of disease is great at all times, enormously great at some. The executive power is sovereign; and, as it is ignorant of medical science, its sovereign act is often directed so as to undermine its own fabric'.[31] William Campbell MacLean, a graduate of Edinburgh who served in the British Army in India, recalled the fatalism of 'authorities, civil and military alike, [who believed that] diseases arose in India, from causes beyond human control; as they could not be "cured", they were to be "endured", and as little said about them as possible'.[32]

Only by acknowledging the authority of medical professionals could the imperial mission be served. Chevers averred that the

> resources of the Physician may do much in anticipating and in relieving disease in detail; but the power of the Law-Giver, if well directed, may do infinitely more in adopting salutary measures which, when properly carried into effect, must materially check the development of large classes of the most destructive maladies...[33]

James Africanus Beale Horton, a West African graduate of Edinburgh University who served in the British West African Army and Colonial Services, predicted a time when a colonial governor would inspire confidence by simply stating that

> my medical officers of health are industriously mapping out the realms of diseases which too often definitely manifest themselves amongst the vilest purlieus of our colonies, and ere long Western Africa [will], I trust, be pronounced one of the healthiest of Her Majesty's inter-tropical possessions since many of the causes of disease are being systematically, energetically, and effectively exterminated by rigid sanitary reform.[34]

By the mid-1880s the indifference of the profession to tropical medicine gave way to gathering interest. Of course, the consolidation of tropical gains after the 'Scramble for Africa' dramatically thrust tropical medicine into the metropolitan consciousness.[35] Yet, as important in the re-making of tropical medicine was overcrowding in the metropolitan profession. Overcrowding and the diminishing opportunity for launching a career in England not only changed attitudes in the profession about imperial appointments, but also sustained interest in tropical medicine.

Multiple forces fuelled the growth of the profession in England after mid-century. First, medicine had long been one of the most direct routes for upward mobility, particularly for Scottish, Irish and English doctors of modest origins. The relative social and economic accessibility of Scottish and later provincial institutions of higher education made university medical degrees more affordable than those from Oxford or Cambridge or London University. Second, the reciprocity provisions of the 1858 Medical Act technically abolished the requirement of a London or English qualification as a condition of eligibility for public positions. As a result, career opportunities were widened for medical men who obtained their professional qualifications in Scotland, Ireland or in the provinces, though the preference for London corporate qualifications remained in force at the leading London teaching hospitals throughout the century.[36] Third, demographic and industrial expansion generated a proliferation of public health legislation and, in turn, numerous public positions for qualified medical men. These developments, together with a public that was anxious about health, improved prospects for a remunerative career in private practice.[37]

Table I
Growth of the Medical Profession in England and Wales, 1861–1901

Date	*Numbers*
1861	14,415
1871	14,692
1881	15,116
1891	19,037
1901	22,698[38]

As Table I shows, the number of doctors in England and Wales remained relatively stable between 1861 and 1881, increasing by only 5 per cent. However, by 1891 the size of the profession surged by 26 per cent and in 1901 by another 19 per cent. Compared to the 26 per cent increase in the size of the employed male population and the 29 per cent increase in the general population between 1861 and 1881, the 5 per cent increase in doctors was small.

Table 2
Doctor-Population (per 1,000) Ratio in England and Wales, 1861–1901

Date	*Ratio*
1861	1,392
1871	1,546
1881	1,718
1891	1,523
1901	1,433[39]

Table 2 illustrates the doctor-population ratio. After a gradual increase in the growth of population to doctors, the ratio dropped after 1881. It could be argued that difference in the ratios, say between 1871 and 1891, is small. But the difference is very significant because the percentage increase in the size of the medical profession from 1891 relative to the increase in the population was far greater than in previous decades.

The surge in the number of doctors surprised census-takers. But, even allowing for the alleged 'misrepresentations' of unqualified doctors, the descriptive evidence from the medical press points to a profession confronting and adjusting to overcrowding.[40] The *Lancet* reported in 1884 that 'the Register shows a steady increase in the number of persons registering annually ... an increase confirmed by the competition in the profession and the obvious excess of practitioners'.[41] A lead article in 1890 noted that 'in every profession there is constantly recurring the cry against overcrowding, and although it is sometimes asserted that the Darwinian principle of the survival of the fittest must tend toward ultimate improvement, this observation lends scant comfort to those who fear being crowded out.'[42]

Of course, fees and income were a constant concern of the profession. But during this period financial prospects appeared to reach an all-time low. E. Paget Thurstan grimly wrote that annual incomes left little for a 'rainy day' and that many doctors faced penury in old age.[43] Head rates for servicing mutual aid societies plunged while the workload increased. One article described such contrasts as 'The Sweating System Applied to the Medical Profession'.[44]

Prospective medical students were advised to reflect on their career decisions. A medical school introductory lecture entitled 'A Few Words of Warning' informed medical students that there was little equity when it came to success. The most earnest failed, and all doctors faced long hours and meagre pay.[45] A notice cautioned parents and young men of 'narrow means' to look elsewhere for an occupation: 'It is strictly true that the medical profession is over-crowded, and cannot be regarded as an eligible "calling" for needy men, or indeed for men who are not practically independent of their work as a means of livelihood.'[46]

Perhaps the most significant index of overcrowding was the new-found interest in imperial appointments. Of interest in the Army Medical Department, Sir Dyce Duckworth candidly observed:

> The 'plums' of civil life are now none too many. Our profession is, in fact, overstocked, and the strife to gain a living in it is very great. Competition is now so keen that some of our humbler brethren are compelled to undertake duties entailing anxiety and serious responsibility for the most miserable remuneration. In times of commercial depression young men are wont to enter our profession, and so, of late years, our ranks have been preternaturally filled.[47]

In spite of the unresolved issue of rank and status, the *Lancet* reported that 'there appears to be no lack of candidates for any branch [the Army, Navy and Indian Service] of public services.'[48] Young doctors were informed that

> all three [services], offer considerable inducements in the way of pay and retirement to young men who may desire to enter at once upon a career in which, from its commencement, they can live on their pay, and have also the right either to retire when they think fit, or to continue to serve with the certainty of a fair pension for life.[49]

In 1889–90 some 50 candidates competed for 12 vacancies in the Colonial Medical Service.[50] A year later, nearly 60 vied for 17 appointments.[51] The *Lancet* conceded that 'though complaints are frequently published in the columns of the *Lancet* of the grievances of colonial surgeons, there always seems to be a sufficient number of candidates for the comparatively small number of such appointments as happens to be vacant'.[52]

George Evatt, an ardent military medical reformer, emphasized overcrowding as a leading factor in the need to organize, that is to professionalize, the Colonial Medical Service 'for the defence of empire'. He wrote:

> No one can to-day look out on the stormy sea of medical professional life without seeing how devoid of organization it is, and how fierce and deadly is the struggle to exist within the profession. Such conditions are as bad for the people and the State as for the physician himself, and call urgently for redress. Afloat on that stormy sea of

> fierce struggle to exist are three or four rafts on which groups of men are struggling to exist in the storm and float to safe-haven to rest. These rafts are the Army Medical Department, the Naval Medical Service, the Indian Medical Service all more or less organized...[53]

Evatt's appeal to empire had a familiar ring. Earlier in the century imperial doctors called for enhancing the social position of medical professionals in the services in the interest of empire. Both prospective and imperial doctors in the latter portion of the century had good reason to be anxious about their position: overcrowding reduced their occupational opportunity and magnified the uneven power relationship between the lay services and medical professionals. No different from their predecessors, medical professionals in the era of the New Imperialism sought to enhance their social position by tying the future empire and the conquest of tropical disease to the reorganization of imperial service.

There was, however, an important distinction between the rhetoric of early and late nineteenth-century proponets of tropical medicine. Before the 1880s imperial doctors rooted their demands for greater professional and service recognition in their occupational knowledge. Later in the century, the metropolitan profession urged reform based on the need to redress the indifference of the 'English' profession to tropical disease. If anything, indifference confirmed the historically low appeal of imperial and colonial service to the metropolitan profession.

As a Scot who served in the Imperial Chinese Customs Service, Patrick Manson's criticism of the parochialism of 'English' pathology is as much a commentary on the limitations of the profession as on the socially constructed nature of tropical medicine. In his Hunterian Society address, Manson declared that 'in our pathology, just as in our politics, as a nation we are too apt to be parochial. In both respects we close our eyes to our imperial position and responsibilities.'[54] He added

> England has wilfully, or rather, ignorantly and indifferently, shut her eyes to one of the biggest facts in pathology revealed during the present century. We seem to have gone to sleep where we ought to have been hard at work and foremost in the ranks of pioneers.[55]

Given the visibility of the new tropical empire, such indifference furnished an opportunity for criticizing and reforming existing institutions, including the imperial services. Imperial doctors who were ideally in the best position to understand and investigate tropical disease lacked training. A leading article in the *British Medical Journal* howled that 'it is not right that a man should be called on to treat disease without having had an opportunity to learn at least something first; and it is not right that the licensing bodies should give the sanction of their degrees to such ignorance'.[56] By the time a surgeon learned to recognize diseases

> ...the energy and enthusiasm of youth have passed, the career in the tropics about over and his health, or his family, or service reasons compel him to leave his work, perhaps just when he was beginning to feel his way to contributing something to the common stock of knowledge.[57]

The situation of doctors in the Indian Medical Service was little better. Ernest Hart, the enterprising editor of the *British Medical Journal,* roundly criticized the paltry research contributions of the Anglo-Indian profession. Hart accused the IMS of discouraging research in an area where England should have been a leader: 'There is a feeling that a man with a leaning to science, with a new scientific fact in his head, is regarded by officialdom as a nuisance, as a sort of pestilent fellow with a new bug.'[58] Seniority and sociability were the keys to a successful career: 'The pathologist is at elbows and is nobody; the diplomatic senior medical officer has all the plums.'[59]

In their proposed reforms both Hart and Evatt emphasized the need for greater attention to medical-scientific research in organizing the Indian and Colonial services. Research into tropical diseases held out tantalizing possibilities for both the British imperial state and the medical professionals. For the former, research would advance the mission of empire and establish Britain's reputation as a leader in a medical-scientific specialty. For the latter, the research imperative would concentrate greater authority and power in medical professionals. In turn, this power would allow doctors to exercise greater control over their function and status in the services.

Hart insisted that research should become a more important criterion in promotion and merit evaluations. Continuing professional education in Europe was to be made available to medical officers of promise. For officers pursuing worthwhile research clerical duties were to be lightened.[60] Evatt called for public, competitive examinations in place of nomination by the Secretary of State. Successful candidates, like Indian and Army officers, would receive specialized instruction at the Army Medical School at Netley. Examinations and/or additional professional qualifications would replace seniority and 'interest' in the distribution of career rewards and promotion.[61]

The campaign to reverse metropolitan indifference to tropical medicine produced no direct improvement in the conditions of imperial service. The profession did take pride in the creation of a lectureship in tropical diseases at St George's Hospital, London, with Patrick Manson as its first occupant.[62] But professional interest in tropical medicine, together with overcrowding in the profession, provided the Colonial Office with ideal conditions to establish the institutional and social basis for supplying its tropical colonies with medical recruits.[63]

Conclusion

It is well known that imperial expansion established the political contours of the problem of tropical disease. Causal agents and prevention and treatment strategies were equally important in defining the significance of tropical disease and health as well. Yet, for far too long historians have unduly relied on the exigencies of the late nineteenth-century tropical empire as an explanation for the transformation of tropical medicine. In so doing, they have totally overlooked the centrality of British medical professionals in the re-making of tropical medicine.

The history of the re-making of tropical medicine is neither a celebration of the corporate influence of the medical profession nor a meditation on the supposed power of medical discourse to transform social reality. Rather, it invites us to reconsider a slightly dated though useful problematic: professionalization. Social status and change in the medical profession both shaped the metropolitan discourse on tropical medicine and diminished the profession's ability to enhance the social position of imperial doctors.

These and other issues of professionalization have continued to shape the specialty well into the present century. Before a meaningful history of tropical medicine can be written, future studies on the imperial services and the scientific specialties that supplanted them need to go beyond the standard administrative and celebratory accounts. Such studies must situate tropical medicine not only in the context of imperialism and colonialism; but also in terms of the social history of medicine and science and British society more generally.

Notes

1. The classic work on this subject is P. D. Curtin, *The Image of Africa: British Ideas and Action, 1780–1850* (Madison: University of Wisconsin Press, 1964). On European mortality and morbidity, see *idem, Death by Migration: Europe's Encounter with the Tropical World in the Nineteenth Century* (Cambridge: University of Cambridge Press, 1991).
2. The literature on the role of medical knowledge in advancing British

imperialism and consolidating colonial British rule continues to grow. For Africa, see L. Spitzer, 'The mosquito and segregation in Sierra Leone', *Canadian Journal of African Studies,* 2 (1968), 49–61; R. Dumett,'The campaign against malaria and the expansion of scientific, medical and sanitary sciences in British West Africa, 1898–1910', *African Historical Studies,* 1 (1968–9); A. Beck, *A History of the British Medical Administration of East Africa, 1900–1950* (Cambridge: Cambridge University Press, 1970); T. S. Gale, 'Official Medical Policy in British West Africa, 1870–1930' (Ph.D. Dissertation, School of Oriental and African Studies, London, 1972); D. R. Headrick, *The Tools of Empire: Technology and European Imperialism in the Nineteenth Century* (Oxford: Oxford University Press, 1981); P. D. Curtin, 'Medical knowledge and urban planning in tropical Africa', *American Historical Review,* 90 (1985), 594–613; J. Cell, 'Anglo-Indian medical theory and the origins of segregation in West Africa', *ibid.,* 91 (1986), 307–35; Megan Vaughan, *Curing their Ills: Colonial Power and African Illness* (Oxford: Oxford University Press, 1991).

3. P. H. Manson-Bahr, *London School of Tropical Medicine, Memoir II: The History of the School of Tropical Medicine in London, 1899–1949* (London: LSTM, 1956); *Liverpool School of Tropical Medicine. Historical Record, 1898–1920* (Liverpool: 1920); D. Fisher, 'Rockefeller Philanthropy and the British Empire: the creation of the London School of Hygiene and Tropical Medicine', *History of Education,* 7 (1978), 129–43; M. Worboys, 'Science and British Colonial Imperialism, 1895–1940.' (D.Phil., Dissertation, University of Sussex, 1979); J. Jones, 'Science, Utility and "Second City of the Empire": the Sciences and Especially the Medical Sciences at Liverpool University, 1881 to 1925' (Ph.D. Dissertation, University of Manchester, 1989).
4. P. H. Manson-Bahr and A. Alcock, *The Life and Work of Patrick Manson* (London: Cassell, 1927); P. H. Manson-Bahr, *The Father of Tropical Medicine* (London: Nelson, 1962); and see note 2.
5. See J. Farley, *Bilharzia: The History of Imperial Tropical Medicine* (Cambridge: Cambridge University Press, 1991); P. Cranefield, *Science and Empire: East Coast Fever in Rhodesia and the Transvaal* (Cambridge: Cambridge University Press, 1991). On the mosquito-filaria hypothesis, see my dissertation 'From the Periphery to the Center: Patrick Manson and the Development of Tropical Medicine as a Medical Specialty in Britain, 1870–1900' (University of California, 1992).
6. M. J. Peterson, *The Medical Profession in Mid-Victorian London* (Berkeley: University of California Press, 1978), 146–7, 197–201 and 204–6. For further discussion, see 'Gentlemen and medical men: The problem of professional recruitment', *Bulletin of the History of Medicine,* 58 (1984), 457–73.

7. For the negotiation between physician and elite patients in diagnosing and treating illness, see N. D. Jewson, 'Medical knowledge and the patronage system in eighteenth-century England', *Sociology*, 8 (1974), 369–85. By the early nineteenth century, however, the medical gaze displaced the patient narrative entirely, see M. E. Fissell, 'The disappearance of the patient's narrative and the invention of hospital medicine' in R. French and A. Wear (eds), *British Medicine in the Age of Reform* (London: Routledge, 1991). Nevertheless, the tension between lay governors and medical professionals in the voluntary hospital continued through the century. See 'Medical officers of hospitals and governors', *Lancet*, 16 August, 1856, 203–4.
8. Peterson, *op. cit.* (note 6). On overcrowding in the early Victorian period and its impact on the profession and on Poor Law medical officers, see I. Loudon, *Medical Care and the General Practitioner, 1750–1850* (Oxford: Oxford University Press, 1986), 208–35.
9. Population of the United Kingdom, 1851–1911 (percentage of total):

	England & Wales	*Scotland*	*Ireland*
1851	65.5	10.5	24.0
1871	72.7	10.7	17.2
1891	76.9	10.7	12.5
1911	79.8	10.5	9.7

Walter L. Arnstein, *Britain Yesterday and Today, 1830 to the Present* (Lexington: 1971), 360.

10. For the Army Medical Department, N. K. Lankford, 'The Victorian medical profession and military practice: army doctors and national origins', *Bulletin of the History of Medicine*, 54 (1980), 528; data on the Indian Medical Service compiled from D. G. Crawford, *Roll of the Indian Medical Service, 1619–1930* (London: Thacker, 1930), 648–9; On the Naval Medical Service, see C. Lloyd and J. L. S. Coulter, *Medicine and the Navy, 1200–1900,* Vol. IV (Edinburgh: 1963), 20. Patterns of geographical mobility for Scottish and Irish medical graduates are also evident in the medical professions of white–settler colonies, see E. B. van Heyningen, 'Agents of Empire: The medical profession in Cape Colony', *Medical History* 33 (1989), 450–71; D. Dyason, 'The medical profession in Colonial Victoria, 1834–1901', in R. MacLeod and M. Lewis (eds), *Disease, Medicine and Empire: Perspectives on Western Medicine and the Experience of European Expansion* (London: Routledge, 1989), 194–216; T. S. Pensabene, *The Rise of the Medical Practitioner in Victoria* (Canberra: Australian National University Press, 1980).
11. Michael Lewis, *The navy in transition* (London: Hodder & Stoughton, 1965): 20–35; E. M. Spiers, *The Army and Society, 1815–1914* (New York, London: Longman, 1980), 1–29.
12. Cited in 'Medical news', *Lancet,* 4 April, 1863, 397.

13. 'The Colonial Medical Service', *ibid.,* 27 May, 1882, 882; also 'Medical practice in Jamaica', *ibid.,* 8 October, 1887.
14. The wrongs of the Army Medical Officers', *ibid.,* 28 March, 1863, 364.
15. For the wrongs of imperial doctors, see J. Bell, *Memorial concerning the Present State of Military and Naval Surgeons to the Right Honourable Earl of Spencer, First Lord of the Admiralty* (Edinburgh: 1808); Anon. *Exposition of the Case of Assistant-Surgeons of the Royal Navy,* 3rd edn, (London: 1850); 'Query', 'The Army Medical Department', *Lancet,* 10 January, 1863, 48; 'Viridis', 'The Army Medical Department', *ibid,* 21 March, 1863, 340; 'Naval Surgeon', 'The Naval Medical Service', *ibid.,* 27 November, 1858, 565–6; 'N. R.', 'The Naval Medical Service', *ibid.,* 15 October, 1859, 399; 'Superceding an Indian Medical Officer', *ibid.,* 28 May, 1859, 546; 'An Ex-Colonial Surgeon', 'Duties and Emoluments of Colonial Surgeons', *ibid.,* 23 July, 1859, 90; 'One Who Has Been Victimised', 'A Warning', *British Medical Journal* (hereafter *BMJ*), 7 March, 1874, 334; 'A British Guiana Surgeon', 'Colonial appointments', *ibid.,* 22 May, 1880, 796; 'The Colonial Medical Service', *ibid.,* 27 May, 1882, 882; 'India and the Colonies: West Africa', *ibid.,* 24 May, 1884, 1019.
16. 'Report of the Committee appointed by the Secretary of State to inquire into the Causes which tend to Prevent Sufficient Candidates from Coming Forward for the Army Medical Department, Parliamentary Papers, XLIV (1878–9), 259–81. Cf. 'Report of the Committee Appointed to Enquire into the Pay, Status, and Conditions of Service of Medical Officers in the Army and Navy', XVII (1889).
17. 'Indian Medical Service', *Lancet,* 21 March, 1863, 335; 'A Deluded Army Surgeon', *ibid.,* 8 August, 1863, 173; 'N.R.', 'The Naval Medical Service', *ibid.,* 15 October, 1859, 399. Against the wishes of army medical officers, composite titles in the army – consisting of both medical and military rank – were abolished in 1886 and replaced by a classified schedule to regulate allowances of all army and departmental officers. See Spiers, *op. cit.* (note 11), 79–80. Naval surgeons found the designation 'assistant surgeon' humiliating. See Anon. *The Exposition of the Case of Assistant-Surgeons of the Royal Navy,* 23. See also 'Report of Commmittee ... into the Causes which tend to Prevent Sufficient Candidates', PP XLVII (1878), 269–72; 'Report of the Committee ... into the Pay, Status, and Conditions of Service of Medical Officers', PP XVII (1889), 142–4; 'Correspondence Relative to the Status of Medical Officers of the Army', PP LC (1890–91), 584–97.
18. 'Medical news: Surgeons for the Army in India', *BMJ,* 10 July, 1858, 571; 'Medical news: No Naval Medical Surgeons', *ibid.,* 27 January, 1866, 109; 'Unpopularity of the Army Medical Department', *Lancet,*

25 July, 1863, 107; 'Breakdown of the Army Medical Department', *BMJ,* 14 May, 1864, 533; 'Notices', 23 February, 1867, 204; 'Unpopularity of the Naval Medical Service', *ibid.,* 25 March, 1871; 'Report of Commitee to Enquire into the Causes that tend to Prevent a Sufficient Number of Candidates'; 'The Medical Service of British Guiana', *BMJ* 7 July, 1883, 26.

19. 'The Admiralty Scheme for Naval Medical Recruits', *BMJ,* 26 January, 1867, 84. See also 'The Army Medical Department', *ibid.'* 4 June, 1864, 616. On the consequences of inadequate pay in the Colonial Medical Service, 'The Colonies', *Lancet,* 22 June, 1878, 914–15.
20. 'Medical News', *ibid.,* 20 February, 1864, 230.
21. See 'Report of Committee Appointed ... to Enquire into the Rank, Pay, and Position of the Medical Officers of the Navy and Army', *Lancet,* 3 March, 1866, 235, 237; 'Navy Medical Department', *ibid.,* 26 March, 1881, 509; 'Why the Indian Service is not popular', *BMJ,* 23 April, 1864, 460; 'The Indian Army Medical Service', *ibid.,* 23 January, 1869, 96; 'Medical education and the Public Services', *ibid.,* 29 April, 1865, 434. 'Return showing the Number of Candidates Examined for Appointments for Indian Medical Department in each year, 1870 to 1879... and similar returns for the Army and Navy Medical Departments', PP LIV (1880), 451–3.
22. On gender, midwives and the medical profession, see J. Donnison, *Midwives and Medical Men: A History of Inter-Professional Rivalries and Women's Rights* (London: 1977); O. Moscucci, *The Science of Women: Gynaecology and Gender in England, 1800–1900* (London: 1990); on tuberculosis and African-Americans, see M. M. Torchia, 'Tuberculosis movement and the race question, 1890–1950', *Bulletin of the History of Medicine,* 49 (1975), 152–95; D. McBride, 'The Henry Phipps Institute, 1903–1937: Pioneering tuberculosis work with an urban minority', *ibid.,* 61 (1987), 78–9; and on gender, race and class in the professionalization of American nursing, see D. C. Hine, *Black Women in White: Racial Conflict and Cooperation in the Nursing Profession, 1890–1950* (Bloomington: Indiana University Press, 1989).
23. 'The Week', *BMJ,* 27 May, 1865, 542–3.
24. *Diseases of Tropical Climates: Lectures Delivered at the Army Medical School* (London: 1886), 3.
25. See 'Medical geography; or, the Geographical Distribution of Health and Disease over the Globe' in W. Aitken *Handbook of the Science and Practice of Medicine* (London: 1862), 727–40. See also C. Hamlin, 'Predisposing causes and public health in early nineteenth-century medical thought', *Journal of the Social History of Medicine,* 5 (1992), 43–70.
26. *Suggestions for the Prevention of that Insidious, and Destructive Foe, to the British Troops in the West Indies, Commonly Termed the Yellow*

Fever (Birmingham: 1808), 7.

27. *A Letter to the Right Honourable, the Secretary of State for War, on Sickness and Mortality in the West Indies, Being a Review of Captain Tulloch's Statistical Report* (London: 1839), 7.
28. *A Manual of Diseases of India, With a Compendium of Diseases* (London: 1886), 3.
29. *A Commentary on the Diseases of India* (London: 1886), 2.
30. 'Presidential Address', *Transactions of the Hong Kong Medical Society* (1889), 1–2.
31. *A Sketch of the History of Febrile Diseases; More Particularly as They Appear in the West Indies Among the Soldiers of the British Army*, 1st edn (London: 1817), xxi.
32. MacLean, *Diseases of Tropical Climates*, 1–2.
33. *A Treatise on Removable and Mitigable Causes of Disease, Their Modes of Origin and Means of Prevention: including a Sketch of the Vital Statistics and Leading Public Health Principles of Public Hygiene in Europe and India* (Calcutta: 1852), 3–4.
34. *Physical and Medical Climate and Metereology of the West Coast of Africa with Valuable Hints to Europeans for the Preservation of Health in the Tropics* (London: 1866), vi–vii.
35. The British empire in Africa grew from 390,574 to 2,496,853 square miles between 1880 and 1895. *The Colonial Office List* (London: 1881 and 1896), 18 and general statistics chart on colonial possessions.
36 B. Haley, *The Healthy Body and Victorian Culture* (Cambridge, Mass.: 1978).
37. 'Report of the Select Committee on the Medical Act Amendment Bills and the Medical Appointments Qualifications Bill with Proceedings, Minute of Evidence', PP, IV (1878–80), 1370–4, 1471–7, 1485–8, 1490–3, 3051–61, 3330–4, 3358–68, 4026–35; 'Report from the Select Committee of the House of Lords on Metropolitan Hospitals', PP, 1890, xvi, 2504–25, 2641–4, 3596–3600, 9042–50, 9706–10; 1890–91, xii, 11, 177–9.
38. These percentages are based on total population in England and Wales and the aggregate number of health professions, including physicians, surgeons and apothecaries. 'Census of England and Wales for 1861, General Report', PP, LIII (1863), Part I, Table I, 247; for 1871, PP, LXXI (1873), Part 2, Appendix A, Table 107, 113; for 1891, CVI (1893–4), 673; 1901 (1904), 92.
39. *Ibid.*
40. See 'Census Report 1891', 673.
41. 'The waste of the medical profession', *Lancet*, 26 July, 1884, 159.
42. 'Overcrowding in the medical profession', *ibid.*, 5 July, 1890, 28.
43. 'Correspondence: A Doctor's Income', *ibid*, 23 April, 1887, 849–59.
44. 'Answers to correspondence: The medical profession and friendly societies', *ibid.*, 5 August,1882, 209; 'Annotations', *ibid.*, 23 March,

1895, 761.

45. 'A Few Words of Warning', *ibid.,* 7 September, 1889, 478.
46. 'Notices: The Medical Profession as a Calling', *ibid.,* 21 February, 1880, 311.
47. 'Valedictory Address', *ibid.,* 10 August,1889 254.
48. 'The Examinations for the Public Medical Services', *ibid.,* 9 February, 1884, 268. The candidate to vacancy ratio was 3 to 1 for the Army, Indian, and Naval Serices.
49. 'The Army, Navy, and Indian Medical Services', *ibid.,* 3 September, 1887, 456.
50. 'Colonial Medical Appointments', *ibid,* 11 April, 1891, 847.
51. 'Medical Appointments in the Colonies', *British Medical Journal,* 4 April, 1891, 770.
52. 'Colonial Appointments' *Lancet,* 11 April, 1891, 847.
53. 'Notes on the Organization of the Colonial Medical Service', *BMJ,* 26 September, 1896, 864.
54. 'Annual Hunterian Address: Malaria, and Its Associated Parasite', *Transactions of the Hunterian Society* (1894–5), 21.
55. *Ibid.*
56. 'Ignorance in Tropical Disease', *BMJ,* 29 December, 1894, 1491–2.
57. *Ibid.*
58. 'An Address on the Medical Profession in India: Its Position and Its Work', *ibid.,* 26 December, 1894, 1474.
59. *Ibid.*
60. *Ibid.*
61. See above, note 53.
62. 'St. George's Hospital', *Lancet,* 6 April, 1895, 885.
63. On the formation of the London School of Tropical Medicine, see my dissertation, chapters 5 and 6.

Index

C

D

F

G

N

THE SCIENCE AND CULTURE OF NUTRITION, 1840-1940

Ed. by Harmke Kamminga and Andrew Cunningham

Amsterdam/Atlanta, GA 1995. 344 pp.
(Clio Medica 32/The Wellcome Institute Series in the History of Medicine)

ISBN: 90-5183-818-2 Bound Hfl. 160,-/US-$ 107.-
ISBN: 90-5183-819-0 Paper Hfl. 50,-/US-$ 33.-

Contents: HARMKE KAMMINGA AND ANDREW CUNNINGHAM: Introduction: The Science and Culture of Nutrition, 1840-1940. HARMKE KAMMINGA: Nutrition for the People, or the Fate of Jacob Moleschott's Contest for a Humanist Science. MARK R. FINLAY: Early Marketing of the Theory of Nutrition: The Science and Culture of Liebig's Extract of Meat. DIETRICH MILLES: Working Capacity and Calorie Consumption: The History of Rational Physical Economy. THOMAS SCHLICH: The Word of God and the Word of Science: Nutrition Science and the Jewish Dietary Laws in Germany, 1820-1920. RINA D. APPLE: Science Gendered: Nutrition in the United States, 1840-1940. L. MARGARET BARNETT: 'Every Man His Own Physician': Dietetic Fads, 1890-1914. MARK WEATHERALL: Bread and Newspapers: The Making of 'A Revolution in the Science of Food'. MIKULÁS TEICH: Science and Food During the Great War: Britain and Germany. SALLY M. HORROCKS: The Business of Vitamins: Nutrition Science and the Food Industry in Inter-war Britain. FERNANDO SALMON: '... but the Patient Remembers the Food': A New Diet, a New Hospital in 1930s Spain. DAVID SMITH AND MALCOLM NICOLSON: Nutrition, Education, Ignorance and Income: A Twentieth-Century Debate. PAUL WEINDLING: The Role of International Organizations in Setting Nutritional Standards in the 1920s and 1930s.

EVOLUTION AND HUMAN VALUES

Ed. by Robert Wesson and Patricia A. Williams

Amsterdam/Atlanta, GA 1995. 251 pp.
(Value Inquiry Book Series 24)
ISBN: 90-5183-830-1 Hfl. 75,-/US-$ 50.-

Initiated by Robert Wesson, *Evolution and Human Values* is a collection of newly written essays designed to bring interdisciplinary insight to that area of thought where human evolution intersects with human values. The disciplines brought to bear on the subject are diverse - philosophy, psychiatry, behavioral science, biology, anthropology, psychology, biochemistry, and sociology. Yet, as organized by co-editor Patricia A. Williams, the volume falls coherently into three related sections. Entitled "Evolutionary Ethics," the first section brings contemporary research to an area first explored by Herbert Spencer. Evolutionary ethics looks to the theory of evolution by natural selection to find values for human living. The second section, "Evolved Ethics," discusses the evolution of language and religion and their impact on moral thought and feeling. Evolved ethics was partly Charles Darwin's subject in *The Descent of Man*. The last section bears the title "Scientific Ethics." A nascent field, scientific ethics asks about the evolution of human nature and the implications of that nature for ethical theory and social policy. Together, the essays collected here provide important contemporary insights into what it is - and what it may be - to be human.
Contributors are: Robert Wesson, Bernard G. Campbell, John H. Campbell, David Depew, Bruce Weber, Howard L. Kaye, Alan Gewirth, Richard J. Herrnstein, Brant Wenegrat, and Patricia A. Williams.

USA/Canada: Editions Rodopi B.V., 2015 South Park Place, Atlanta, GA 30339, Tel. (770) 933-0027, *Call toll-free* (U.S. only) 1-800-225- 3998, Fax (770) 933-9644, *E-mail:* F.van.der.Zee@rodopi.nl

All Other Countries: Editions Rodopi B.V., Keizersgracht 302-304, 1016 EX Amsterdam, The Netherlands. Tel. + + 31 (0)20-622-75-07, Fax + + 31 (0)20-638-09-48, *E-mail:* F.van.der.Zee@rodopi.nl